AF531612

# Beyond the Milk Pail

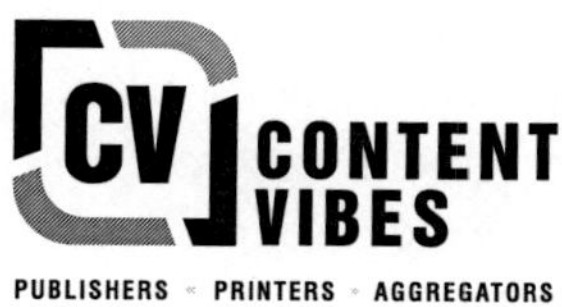

## About the Authors

**Ms. Chimi Yangzom Lepcha** is currently pursuing her Ph.D. in the Division of Agricultural Extension at ICAR-Indian Agricultural Research Institute (ICAR-IARI) in New Delhi, India. She earned her B.Sc. in Agriculture from the College of Agriculture, Pasighat, under Central Agricultural University, Imphal, and her M.Sc. in Agricultural Extension from ICAR-NDRI. Ms. Lepcha has qualified for prestigious fellowships such as the ICAR-JRF/SRF and UGC-NET Junior Research Fellowship (JRF). Additionally, she passed the National Eligibility Test (NET) conducted by ASRB in 2022 in Agricultural Extension, which qualifies her for Lecturership/Assistant Professorship. Her academic contributions include a range of research articles, book chapters, and popular articles in various journals. She is also actively involved in seminars, conferences, workshops, and training programs, demonstrating her commitment to advancing the field of agricultural extension.

**Dr. Asif Mohammad** is working as Senior Scientist in the section of Dairy Extension at ERS of ICAR-NDRI. He got 'Amitabha Mukherjee Gold Medal' for securing first class first position in B.Sc. (Ag.) of Visva Bharati University. He obtained M.Sc. and Ph.D. from ICAR-National Dairy Research Institute. He got 'Director's Gold Medal' for securing first class first position in Management group of ICAR- National Dairy Research Institute. Dr. Mohammad received advanced long duration training from Asian Institute of Technology, Pathum Thani, Thailand. He has published more than 50 research papers in reputed national and international journals. He has more than 14 years of experience in extension research, teaching and field demonstrations. He has expertise in organizing structured training programmes and evaluation of effectiveness of training and capacity building programmes. He is expert in the field of impact assessment and social system analysis. He has good experience in psychometric scale construction techniques and development of index relevant for social science studies.

**Mr. Bikram Barman** is a Ph.D. Research Scholar in the Division of Agricultural Extension at ICAR-Indian Agricultural Research Institute (ICAR-IARI), New Delhi, India. He completed his B.Sc. in Agriculture from Uttar Banga Krishi Viswavidyalaya, Majhian campus, West Bengal and his M.Sc. in Agricultural Extension from ICAR-NDRI. He qualified for the ICAR-JRF/SRF and UGC-NET Junior Research Fellowship (JRF). Additionally, he passed the National Eligibility Test (NET) conducted by ASRB in 2023 in the Discipline of Agricultural Extension for Lecturership / Assistant Professorship eligibility. His contributions include several research articles, book chapters, and popular articles published in various national journals. His active participation in numerous seminars, conferences, workshops, and training programs underlines his dedication to the field.

**Dr. Girish C E** completed his Ph.D. from the Eastern Regional Station of ICAR-National Dairy Research Institute (NDRI) in Kalyani. His academic journey began with a B.Sc. in Agriculture from the College of Agriculture in Mandya, under the University of Agricultural Sciences, Bengaluru. He was a recipient of the prestigious Junior Research Fellowship from ICAR, which enabled him to pursue his M.Sc. in Agricultural Extension Education at ICAR-NDRI. His academic excellence continued as he was awarded the NDRI-Institute fellowship during his Ph.D. studies. In 2023, he qualified for the National Eligibility Test (NET) conducted by the Agricultural Scientists Recruitment Board (ASRB) in the discipline of Agricultural Extension for Assistant Professorship eligibility. His research contributions are significant, with numerous research papers and popular articles published in various esteemed journals. His achievements and contributions to Agricultural Extension highlight his dedication and expertise in the field.

# Beyond the Milk Pail
## Multidimensional Insights into Women's Participation in Dairy Farming in East Sikkim

**Chimi Yangzom Lepcha**
Division of Agricultural Extension
ICAR-Indian Agricultural Research Institute (ICAR-IARI)
New Delhi, India

**Asif Mohammad**
Eastern Regional Station
ICAR- National Dairy Research Institute
Kalyani, West Bengal, India

**Bikram Barman**
Division of Agricultural Extension
ICAR-Indian Agricultural Research Institute (ICAR-IARI)
New Delhi, India

**Girish C E**
Eastern Regional Station
ICAR- National Dairy Research Institute
Kalyani, West Bengal, India

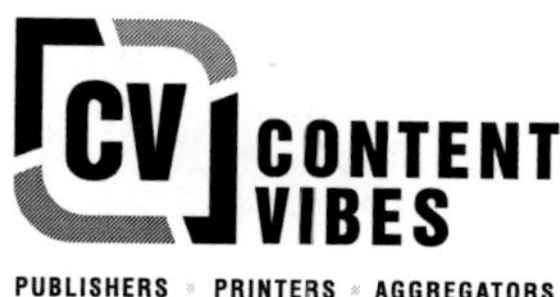

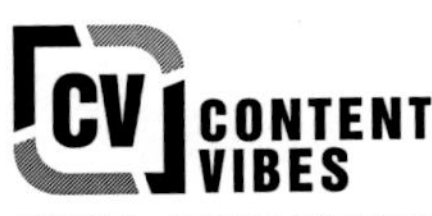


1168, Sector 13, Urban Estate
Karnal-132 001, Haryana
Tel: 91-84470 75807, 18440 41168
Email: contentvibesppa@gmail.com
www.contentvibes.in



Print ISBN: 978-81-97719-20-2
ebook-ISBN: 978-81-97719-23-3

# Perface

While the critical role of women in agriculture, particularly dairy farming, is undeniable, their contributions often go unnoticed. This is especially true in East Sikkim, where women's tireless efforts are vital to the sustenance of both households and communities. This book seeks to bridge this knowledge gap by providing a comprehensive analysis of women's roles and contributions within this region's dairy sector. Through meticulous research, this book delves into the daily activities, decision-making processes, and challenges faced by these women. It offers a nuanced understanding of their significant, yet under-acknowledged, contributions. By examining their work routines, involvement in key decisions, and the obstacles they encounter, we aim to shed light on the indispensable role of women in dairy farming.

This work will be a valuable resource for students, researchers, policymakers, and anyone interested in agricultural development and gender equity in farming. It provides a foundation for understanding the intricate dynamics of women's participation in the dairy sector and highlights areas where support and intervention are needed to enhance their contributions and well-being.

We extend our sincere gratitude to the Director of ICAR-NDRI, the Head of ERS of ICAR-NDRI, our respondents, and the numerous sources that have enriched this book. Their support and insights have been instrumental in bringing this research to fruition. We trust this work will illuminate the indispensable role of women in dairy farming and contribute to their empowerment, fostering greater recognition and appreciation of their efforts within the agricultural sector and beyond.

**Chimi Yangzom Lepcha**
**Asif Mohammad**
**Bikram Barman**
**Girish C E**

# Contents

# List of Tables

# List of Maps

# List of Figures

# List of Plates

# 1

# Introduction

*"I measure the progress of a community by the degree of progress which women have achieved"*

***–B. R. Ambedkar***

India is one of the most populous country in the world with a population of 1.26 billion (Census,2011). Of which women constitute about 49 percent of the population. Women act as a significant factor in development of the nation. Women from all sphere of life are contributing meaningly towards the prosperity of the nation. Especially, the rural farm women who constitute nearly half of the total rural population. The rural women are the mainstay of Indian agriculture. Their contribution towards agriculture development is worthy of praises. They are capable of accomplishing sustainable development in all the various activities which they have carried out and shown interest. Women are the essential part of society. For a society to develop, women should be given equal importance as the male counterpart. Nurturing of society is possible only if women are nurtured with equivalent opportunities and progress. Indian society is still male dominant, which accounts for low reputation of women. Women are treated as less competent human being. Through passing of time there have been acknowledgement by the Constitution of India on the part of importance of women as a productive humane resource for development of nation. Many measures have been adopted for the gender equality. This paved the way for advancement of empowerment of women. Kabeer (1999), classified measurement of empowerment into resources, agency and achievements, where resources are conceptualized as having hold over bodily, financial and human rational resources, agency is conceptualized as ability to make their own choices and achievements refers to combination of resources and agency, related to ultimate functioning and individual penchants. Economic opportunity of women in India is actively changing its trend towards upward direction. The women work force is increasing, predominantly in professional field, which is setting a benchmark. Despite of these changes, there are still number of women who act as invisible worker in unorganized sector. Rural women are mostly deprived from many facilities like education and training due to their rural background, caste, cultural practices and socio-economic condition. The urban and upper-class women are entering the work force and establishing themselves in all the fields.

## 1.1 Women's role in agriculture

Agriculture is an important sector in the country which promote economic development of the nation. In India, nearly 70 percent of the population lives in rural village and 60 percent of population is engaged in agriculture and its allied activities to earn a livelihood (Rao, 2006). Agriculture sector provides employment facilities to the rural population and boost the economy of the nation. Majority of rural women depends on agriculture for sustaining their livelihood. Women constitutes about 33 percent of total agriculture cultivator and about 47 percent of total agriculture labour, (Rao, 2006). Farm women are the integral part of agriculture. They perform multiple roles in agriculture and allied sector. In developing countries like ours, women are accountable for production of 60 to 80 percent of food production (FAO,2011). Farm women performs various labour-intensive work in agriculture like, weeding of the field, ploughing of small land, sowing of crop, harvesting of the crop, storage etc. According to FAO (2011), the time contributed by the women in agriculture activities was estimated to be 32 percent.

## 1.2 Role of women in dairy farming

Under the agriculture and allied sector, livestock sector plays an important role in securing livelihood of rural population. Dairying is one such activity which bring significant change in socio- economic condition of the rural poor. India holds the first position in milk production in the world with 187.7 MT milk production during 2018-19 (DAHDF,2019). Thus, dairy is one of the major contributors of livelihood security for the rural people, especially for rural farm women. The dairy enterprise is believed to be a boon to the Indian economy. It has the potential to generate extra income, which is attracting many rural populations, particularly the farm women to adopt the dairy farming. The farm women contribute significantly to the dairy related activities. The activities performed by the rural women in livestock management mostly include watering the animals, care of new born calf and sick animals, making of cow dung cake and their disposal (Bose *et al.*, 2013). The farm women participation was found to be highest in cleaning of animal shed, feeding, cleaning of animals and least in marketing aspect of the animal produce and animal grazing (Javed *et al.*, 2006). Many studies have shown that the rural women earn extra income from sale of milk and animals. Their participation in dairy farming resulted in decrease in poverty and increase in standard of living.

## 1.3 Status of dairy farming in India

According to the 20th livestock census (2019), the total livestock population in the country is 536.76 million which has shown 4.60 percent of increase over the last census. The total livestock in the country is 11.54 percent. The exotic/crossbred cattle population in the country is 51.36 million which increased by 29.30 percent and indigenous cattle population is 142.11 million, respectively. The exotic/crossbred milch cattle increased by 34.30 percent and indigenous milch cattle has increased by 0.80 percent than the previous census period. States like Uttar Pradesh, Rajasthan, Madhya Pradesh and West Bengal are having the highest number of livestock population. India is one of the top most milk producing countries in the world. Milk production in the country during 1991-92 was 55.6 million tonnes and in 2018-19 it was 187.7 million tonnes (DAHD&F,2019). The per capita milk availability was 394gms/day in 2018-19. The dairy sector has proved to be an integral subordinate source of income for the rural families in the country for sustaining the livelihood. Mostly the milk produced by the animals in the country is nurtured by small and marginal dairy farmers. In India, 48.00 percent of the total milk produced is consumed at the producer level while the 52.00 percent is marketable surplus, out of which 40.00 percent of milk is taken by the organised sector and the 60.00 percent is taken by the unorganised sector. The total number of women engaged in dairy cooperatives in the country was about 4.9 million. The total number of women dairy cooperative society (DCS) was 32,092, which involved 29.50 percent of the total farmers as on 31.03.2018(DAHD&F).

## 1.4 Dairying in Sikkim

In Sikkim, dairy farming has been a traditional practice of the rural population for generating economic security. Sikkim being a mountainous state, livestock rearing holds a vital role in maintaining the livelihood activities in the region. Animal husbandry sector acts as a major source of additional income for the rural people of Sikkim (Bhasin, 1995). In Sikkim, the population with higher economic status have no involvement in the agriculture activities when compared with the lower economic status population. Animal husbandry is seen as a predominantly female oriented enterprise for medium and low economic strata of society. The farm women act as strong pillar in the state for dairy development. On an average woman work 3.5 hours per day for the animal husbandry activities and men works for only 1.6 hours per day (Verma, 1992). The milk production in the state during 2017-18 was 58.67 tonnes. The availability of per capita milk in the state was 244 gm/day (2017-18). Number of organized Dairy Cooperative Societies (DCS) was 497. The number of farmers members enrolled under DCS was 13687. Average milk procurement by DCS was 36 TKgPD which involves 22.40 percent of total milk production. State has 14 number of bulk milk coolers with capacity of 9 thousand litres per day (TLPD) and number of processing plants in the state were 3 with capacity of 60 TLPD (State Dairy Profiles, 2019). According to the 20$^{th}$ livestock census (2019), total number of livestock population in the state was 391,110. The exotic/ crossbred cattle population in the state was 116,850 and the population of indigenous cattle was 148,010.

### 1.5 Statement of problem

Dairying in India has been a women centric enterprise. Women farmers act as a key player in livestock activities, in inclusion to their daily household chores. Gender equity is more established in dairy related activities compared to other sectors, where women comprise of approx. 69 percent of the work force. In India participation of women engaged in dairying is about 75 million compared to 15 million men (Thakur and Chander, 2006). However, the women's contribution is not recognised as dairy worker. Farm women are seen as a covert worker. Their contribution to the dairy related activities is often scantly acknowledged as these activities are not determined in profit- making term. There are fewer evidences about the engagement of women in dairy market chain, showing lesser role in the market related aspect. Farm women of East district of Sikkim are practicing dairy farming as a means to earn a livelihood. Most of the decision-making aspect regarding the dairying are taken by the male counterparts. The farm women usually performed tedious work in dairying, like cleaning of cattle shed, collection of feed and fodder etc. Women are unduly represented as unpaid, seasonal and part-time worker in agriculture activities. Many studies have shown that women are paid in lesser amount compared to the men in the same work. Gender stereotype about men as farmer and female as housewives resulted in the influence of perception of people about the role of women in dairy activities. The contribution of the women in agriculture has been known, but the exact intensity of the contribution in terms of magnitude and nature is often difficult to assess. There are many constrains faced by the farm women in dairying that is, inadequate knowledge about breed, timely health management operation, high cost of feed and fodder, lack of training facility etc which are hampering the performances and empowerment of farm women. There is a need to recognize the contribution made by women in the dairy sector, which in turn will help in empowerment of women to hold a greater position in this sector. The participation of the women in dairy sector has to be understood rightly, to predict the future role of women. There is also a need to correct the gender biasness and different constrains faced by the farm women should be identified through feedback from dairy women farmer. The purpose of the study is to acquire adequate knowledge in the differential role accomplished by the farm women in the dairy related activities, to estimate the socio-economic empowerment of the women in dairy farming and to analyse the feedback of the women engaged in dairying in the state of Sikkim.

According to the problem discussed above, research questions were formulated to offer solution and those problems are written as follows:

1. Whether there is any significant difference in role performed by the women in dairying from different social strata in East district of Sikkim?
2. What is the magnitude of socio-economic empowerment of women engaged in dairying?
3. What are the factors linked with the participation of women in dairying?

Therefore, the study entitled **Beyond the Milk Pail: Multidimensional Insights into Women's Participation in Dairy Farming in East Sikkim** with the specific objectives has been proposed:

## Objectives

1. To assess the differential role accomplished by women dairy farmers from different social strata in the study area
2. To measure the magnitude of socio-economic empowerment of women dairy farmer of the study area
3. To analyze the feedback of women engaged in dairying

## 1.6 Justification of the study

The study is focussed to assess the differential role of women in the dairy farming from different social strata in the East district of Sikkim. This will result in bringing attention to different work carried out by the women in the dairy sector. This study will provide in-depth understanding about the women's role in the present which in turn will help in formulating the future role. This will help the researchers in getting comprehensive knowledge about the role of women in dairy. The study will also help in highlighting the work load difference between the women in various economic strata in the state. This study is intended to find the empowerment of dairy farm women in terms of socio- economic condition. The socio-economic empowerment measure will help to know about the status of women in the society, their standard of living and the quality and quantity of capacity building required for skill development of the farm women to achieve gender equality in the society. Getting the idea regarding the women's role and their contribution, the study will help to identify different factors affecting women's participation and to highlight the roadmap to encourage active participation of women in dairy sector of Sikkim. This study will contribute to the social science research in the state of Sikkim, which is inadequate regardless of several incentives provided by the state government.

## 1.7 Scope of the study

1. The result of the present study would intensify the knowledge about the differential role performed by the women dairy farmers of the East district of Sikkim with respect to their social strata.
2. The study would help in development of roadmap for empowerment of the dairy women by measuring the magnitude of empowerment with respect to socio-economic variables.
3. The study would throw light on the various feedback given by the women dairy farmers, which could help the policy maker in identifying the felt need and problem faced by the women dairy farmers, for chalking out suitable developmental schemes for women dairy farmers.
4. The study could be of immense help to the government officials in framing strategies for development of dairy sector, provide several opportunities to the dairy farmers and implementing useful schemes related to women dairy farmers.

## 1.8 Limitation of the study

1. Limited amount of time and resources were available to the researcher to conduct the study in the state of Sikkim was one of the major shortcomings. Hence, the researcher has put on full effort to make the study systematic and objective specific.
2. This study involved face to face interaction with the respondent regarding issues like their role in dairy farming, empowerment and feedback given by them, their responses might be recalled information which may lead to some random errors.
3. The study did not guarantee the responses obtained from the respondent is free from any bias or prejudice.
4. This study could not be generalized as it is confined to a particular area only.
5. Limited number of variables had been considered under the study due to limited resources and time.

## 1.9 Organization of Book

The book is divided into five chapters in a systematic manner. The first chapter is “Introduction” which includes some basic information about the role of women in agriculture and dairying and the dairy status in India and Sikkim, statement of problem, objectives of the study, scope of study and limitation of the study. The second chapter is "Review of literature", where reviews about the past literature has been provided. "Research Methodology" chapter is the third chapter which includes locale of study, sampling plan, operationalization of variables. The fourth chapter is "Results and Discussion" which includes the main findings of the study and discussion of found results. The fifth chapter is the "Summary and Conclusions" where suggestions are given. Bibliography is presented at the end.

# 2

# Review of Literature

Research being a continuous process for a scientific study, previous study provides basis for the research. The review of literature is necessary for developing conceptual frame work and suitable design for the study. It assists the researcher to keep his work going in right direction. The available literature related to the present study has been reviewed under the following heading:

## 2.1 Differential role accomplished by women dairy farmers from different social strata

Toppo *et al.* (2004) examined the participation of women farmers in dairy occupation in Anand district of Gujarat and their result revealed that 18.34 percent of the farm women were mostly engaged in activities related to artificial insemination, majority of the respondent (68.34%) participated in cleaning of the shed, while 25.00 percent of the farm women practised manure preparation and 95.00 percent of the respondent were not involved in preparation of gobar gas mixture.

Badole (2006) reported that majority of the responded had low socio-economic status.

Tayde (2006) examined the farm women empowerment in Marathwada region of Maharashtra and found that 14.15 percent of the respondent belonged to Scheduled Tribe/NT/SBC category, 17.50 percent belonged to Other Backward Caste category, 33.34 percent to Open caste and 35.00 percent were found to be Scheduled Caste category.

Younas *et al.* (2007) examined the work carried out by the farm women in dairy activities in Punjab and revealed that rural women were spending almost 15 hours a day in dairy related activities and out of which 5 to 6 hours were spend on caring for livestock cattle.

Sharma (2008) studied the socio- economic status of farm women and the study revealed that majority of the farm women had medium socio- economic status.

Narmatha *et al.* (2009) found that majority of farm women performed actual work in management of livestock, followed by feeding, health care and breeding but participated less in marketing, insurance activity and maintenance of record.

Chauhan (2011) reported that tribal farm women of Gujarat were engaged in collection of feed and fodder, feeding of cattle, cleaning of cattle and cattle shed, milking, preparation of milk products, taking animal for grazing and veterinary services. The farm women were active in taking decision regarding the animal husbandry activity.

Kaur *et al.* (2011) conducted research on measurement of empowerment of the rural women and revealed that majority (59.00%) of the farm women were found to be from backward caste.

Rathod *et al.* (2011) reported that farm women were the main performer in small scale dairy farming. They were responsible for all the critical activities related to dairy but had low participation in decision making regarding the sale and purchase related to dairy.

Khan *et al.* (2012) conducted their study on women's participation on agriculture activities in the Peshawar district and revealed that on an average the farm women were spending 6.23 hours on livestock related activities on daily basis and 1.09 hours on selling of milk.

Bhanotra *et al.* (2015) revealed the role of rural women in decision making in livestock management in Kathua district of Kashmir. Result revealed that women mostly participated in taking care of new born calf, sick animals, feeding of animals and cleaning activities and less participation in breeding, sale of animal and cultivation of fodder crops.

Kaur (2015) found that 26.60 percent of the farm women were efficiently involved in obtaining loans from the institutional sources while 12.00 percent of the farm women were involved in maintaining financial records of their dairy farm and majority of the respondents belonged to low income category.

Upadhyay and Yadav (2015) conducted their research in Bhilwara district of Rajasthan where they studied the socio-economic profile of 240 women dairy farmer and found that majority (45.42%) of the farm women belonged to Other Backward Classes (OBC), whereas 39.58 percent belonged to general and 11.25 percent belonged to Scheduled Caste and only 3.75 percent belonged to Scheduled Tribe.

Yasmin and Ikemoto (2015) studied women's participation in small scale dairy farming for poverty reduction and signified that farm women managed the dairy farming activities. Their participation in economic activities increased after practising small scale dairy farming.

Jahan and Khan (2016) conducted their study on farm women's participation in animal husbandry and revealed that, 95.50 percent of the respondent had participated in collection and chaffing of the fodder, 99.00 percent of them were engaged in milking of the cattle, 93.00 percent in taking care of the health of the cattle, 88.50 percent in preparation of cow dung cakes and maintaining the hygiene of the shed and 62.50 percent were involved in marketing of milk and milk products.

Kavithaa and Rajkumar (2016) studied the decision-making behaviour of farm women in dairy farming activities in Erode district of Tamil Nadu and found that farm women were dominant in taking decision regarding activities which does not involve financial aspect like taking care of new born, sick and pregnant animal, milking, processing of milk and making use of the dung and were less dominant in making decision regarding economic aspect.

Patel *et al.* (2017) examined the socio -economic profile of dairy farm women in Junagadh district of Gujarat and reported that least respondent belonged to Scheduled Tribe (6.00 %) followed by Scheduled Caste (16.50 %), majority of the respondent belonged to Other Backward Caste (44.00 %) while rest of the respondents belonged to General (33.50 percent) category and also studied the participation of farm women in decision making regarding dairy farming in Junagadh district of Gujarat and reported that majority of respondent were taking active decision on milking, milk products processing and milch cattle management

Kaur *et al.* (2019) studied the participation appraisal of women farmers in dairy husbandry practices in Indo-Pak border area of Punjab (India) and reported that majority of the respondent were from General category (83.13%) followed by Scheduled Caste, 10.63 percent and Others, 6.25 percent. The study also showed that over all participation of farm women in animal husbandry practices and revealed that majority of the respondent (70.00%) had medium participation followed by 16.87 percent had low participation and 13.13 percent had high participation respectively.

Dash *et al.* (2020) studied the role of dairy cooperative society in empowering women in rural Odisha, reported that 40.00 percent of the respondents belonged to Other Backward Caste while, 30.60 percent belonged to Scheduled Caste and 29.40 percent belonged to General category. In terms of economic status, 74.60 percent respondents belonged to below poverty line (BPL) and 25.40 percent of the respondents belonged to above poverty line (APL), respectively.

Kaur and Kaur (2021) revealed that farm women were performing all the dairy activities. In the case of small farm size, women dairy farmers were more actively participating in all the activities related to dairy farming while in the case of large farm size, women dairy farmers were heiring labour for carrying out the activities due to large number of dairy cattle and they had sufficient income in their household. They also reported that dairy farm women had no independence in decision making.

From the above reviews it is clearly understood that farm women were taking active participation in dairy related activities. Their roles in the dairy sector are crucial for the sustaining the livelihood of their family.

## 2.2 Magnitude of socio-economic empowerment of women dairy farmer

Gunjkar (2005) revealed that 74.67 percent of the respondent had no social empowerment.

Kamalkannan and Namasivayam (2005) revealed that economic empowerment was conceivable only if the women had full control over their income and resources. Entrepreneurship activities among women can be the probable way towards economic empowerment.

Sudhindra (2005) examined the empowerment through watershed development in Kolar district of Karnataka and concluded that, women who were the member of self help group were more empowered, they were financially sound and paid the debts through their saving and were engaged in activities like rearing of goats and selling of milk and milk products.

Sampat (2008) revealed that after joining the self help group 72.50 percent of the farm women had high level of economic empowerment, 95.83 percent of the farm women had high social empowerment and 98.33 percent of the respondents had high cultural empowerment.

Tayde and Chole (2010) studied empowerment appraisal of rural women and reported that in social empowerment, majority of the women had the freedom to mingle with the social female groups but were restricted to visit the clinics and hospital, while in economical empowerment the women enjoyed all the freedom related to the aspect of economic empowerment dimensions other than decision related to marketing of produce, having a saving in fixed deposit and heiring labours.

Sajesh *et al.* (2011) reported that SHG had a significant influence on empowerment of rural women.

Shambharkar *et al.* (2012) revealed that after the participation of women in SHG, majority of the women had the access to the financial transaction and there was no sign of insufficient power among the women after being the member of SHG. Three fifth (61.43%) of the respondents had medium empowerment level and only 0.71 percent respondents had low empowerment level.

Damodar and Rathod (2013) studied the influence of Mahila Arthik Vikas Mahamandal, MAVIM activities on empowerment of rural women in Nagpur district of Maharashtra and revealed that after the women's involvement in the MAIVM activities, majority of the farm women had overall high level of empowerment.

Shiralashetti (2013) concluded that economic empowerment was responsible for increase of women's approach towards economic assets, job opportunities, financial assistance, valuable possession, capacity building and marketing information.

Islam *et al.* (2014) signified the importance of microcredit on women's empowerment in rural Bangladesh. Dimensions like economic and household decision-making, mobility, property ownership, and social awareness were used in measuring the empowerment. Their results revealed that the microcredit program led to the improvement in empowerment of the women. It had a positive relation with the given dimension of empowerment.

Jadav *et al.* (2014) reported that training of the women in dairy related activities had a crucial role in empowerment of farm women and revealed that farm women who were trained were more active and quicker in adopting new technology and being empowered than the untrained farm women.

Kadam *et al.* (2014) examined the empowerment of women through SHGs and revealed that, 36.67 percent of the women of the SHG had medium level of empowerment, 18.33 percent of the SHG women had high level of empowerment and about 15.58 percent of the respondent had low level of empowerment. It was also reported that the profile of the women member of SHGs had a positive and significant relation with the empowerment.

Tekale *et al.* (2014) reported that, 86.00 percent of the respondent had the freedom of choosing of jobs, 73.00 percent had the power to give employment to labourers, 69.00 percent made decision regarding adoption of the modern technologies, 60.00 percent had ability to purchase inputs for family, 58.00 percent had personal bank accounts,53.00 percent had saving in fixed deposit and 51.00 percent involved in decision making of marketing of the produce.

Damodar *et al.* (2016) reported the relationship of personal, socio-economic and situational characteristics with the empowerment of rural women. The study revealed that variables like education, land holding, caste, income of the family had a significant relation with the overall empowerment while extension participation, type of family, age and size of family were not significant in explaining the overall empowerment.

Basha (2017) studied the empowerment of women through SHG and the study described that SHG resulted in financial improvement of the farm women by generating additional income and empowering them.

Patel *et al.* (2017) signified the involvement of farm women in dairy and reported that majority of the respondent (47.00%) had low level of social participation whereas, 46.00 percent of respondent had medium level of social participation and only 7.00 percent had high social empowerment.

Das *et al.* (2019) signified that education, land, house type, material possessed, family income, social participation, mass media exposure, training, monetary benefits etc were having a significant relationship with the empowerment. The study also showed the path analysis and found that socio-economic status was having highest direct effect on empowerment whereas income of the family was having highest indirect effect on empowerment.

Islam *et al.* (2019) studied the women's empowerment through small scale dairy farming in Bangladesh and found that through the small-scale dairy farming women were able to make decision regarding household and personal care, gained self-confidence.

Hasan *et al.* (2020) found that women in Bangladesh were very less empowered in taking decision regarding the agriculture and livestock activities while they were empowered in taking decision regarding non- agriculture activities.

Dash *et al.* (2020) studied the role of dairy cooperative society in empowering women in rural Odisha and reported that after the farm women joined the dairy cooperative their economic empowerment increased as a result of their increase in income and there was increase in social empowerment as the social status was enhanced after joining the dairy cooperative. They also reported that women dairy cooperative society had significant influence on financial state of farm women.

The Self-Help Groups, dairy cooperatives played an important role in creating awareness about the empowerment in women farmers. High literacy rate, active participation in social activities, access to credit, ability to take decision were some aspects of women empowerment

## 2.3 Feedback given by women engaged in dairying

Yadav and Sethi (2000) reported that, lack of communication in spreading of the important messages related to the dairy technology was seen in the rural areas. Thus, they suggested the use of media for efficient communication of the messages to the farm women so that they can get useful information regarding dairy technology.

Chinnadurai *et al.* (2002) examined farm women in commercial dairy farming and found that low rate of milk price, limited availability of green fodder around the year, inadequate financial resources and transport facility were some problems faced by the farm women.

Agrawal *et al.* (2007) revealed that, 92.00 percent of the dairy farm women had inadequate progeny tested bulls, 84.00 percent respondents had unavailability of high yielding fodder variety, 78.00 percent of respondents crossbred cattle had low fat content, 67.00 percent faced high mortality in young crossbred males.

Kale *et al.* (2013) revealed that cost of concentrate feed was high, the farm women had inadequate finance to buy crossbred animals and medicines, also the performance of the exotic breed was declining due to the summer temperature. Overall, the farm women had little knowledge about the scientific dairy management.

Upadhyay *et al.* (2013) analysed some constrictions of the dairy farm women in animal husbandry and reported some aspect like expensive concentrate feed, scanty knowledge about the animal husbandry practices, deficiency of roughages, non- remunerative milk prices and limited training facility on dairy activities were some problems faced by dairy farm women.

Patel *et al.* (2016) reported some major problems faced by the dairy farm women which were as follows, low remunerative price for milk, lack of skilled labour, insufficient cheap green fodder round the year, inadequate concentrate feed, lack of knowledge about scientific cattle management.

Sadashive *et al.* (2016) conducted study on "constraints faced by the dairy farmers in running dairy enterprises", and revealed that limitations like insufficiency of drinking water, unavailability of feed and fodders, low conception rate, lack of housing facility for animal, incidence of disease and poor price of milk, were the major restraints faced by the respondent.

Chakravarthi *et al.* (2017) revealed some limitations confronted by the dairy farmers in Kadapa district of Andhra Pradesh; those were insufficient knowledge about disease control and ration balancing, high cost of construction and non-remunerative price for milk.

Panchbhai *et al.* (2017) reported some restraints met by dairy farmers were low productivity of the cattle (92.50%), costly cross bred animals (89.00%), costly concentrate fodder (87.00%), (78.00%) insufficient knowledge about scientific milking practices and lack of knowledge about disease and vaccination (67.00%).

Prasad *et al.* (2017) reported major limits faced by dairy farmers which was low price for milk, recurring disease breakout like mastitis, non-availability of feed and fodder all year round.

Pathade *et al.* (2017) analysed the limitations faced by the SHG women involved in dairy farming. The result revealed that conception rate through artificial insemination (AI) was found to be low, the productivity of local breeds was poor, timely payment from dairy cooperatives was delayed and far off location of milk collection centres were the major shortcomings, that the farm women had to undergo.

Niketha *et al.* (2018) examined the problems faced by the members of women dairy cooperatives in Karnataka and found that farm women considered illiteracy as major personal constraints. Farm women had low support from the family in participation in culture and social activities. Diversified workload, lack of interest in handling technical gadgets was some problem faced by the farm women.

Sharma *et al.* (2018) reported that farm women of Nainital district were facing mostly problem regarding breeding disorder of the milch cattle, access for market input was limited, disease and pest infestation, lack of availability of concentrate feed and mineral mix, insufficient knowledge about the scientific dairy practices etc.

Dhayal *et al.* (2020) studied some major constraints perceived by the tribal farm women and found some major constraints were migration for labour during different seasons, low literacy rate of the tribal women, poor economic condition and their shy nature.

From the above reviews some major problems which was taken as a feedback given by the farm women were, were lack of green fodder round the year, no remunerative prices for milk, high price of concentrate, feed and fodders, lack of knowledge about credit schemes and proper veterinary services.

## Gaps in knowledge

1. Scanty research on assessing the differential role performed by the farm women in dairying pertaining to their different social strata in the state.
2. Limited effort has been taken to study about the socio- economic empowerment of the farm women whose livelihood is mostly generated through dairy farming in the state of Sikkim.
3. Limited analysis of the field data on the social science research and feedback from the farm women engaged in dairy farming in Sikkim.

# 3

# Research Methodology

Research methodology gives detailed justification about the research methods and procedures carried out in the present study. The present study focuses on the women's involvement in the dairy farming and their empowerment. Keeping in view the specific objectives of the study and various aspects relating to these objectives the methodological framework has been formulated. The sub topic under the research methodology is as follow:

## 3.1 Locale of the study

The present study entitled **"Retrospective Multidimensional Study on Magnitude of Participation of Women in Dairy Farming in East district of Sikkim"** was carried out in the villages of East district of Sikkim. Sikkim is the second smallest states in India, with an area of 7,096 sq. km in size. The meaning of Sikkim is "The valley of rice". It lies between 27 °33' 00" N and 88 °30' 00" E. The average annual temperature of the state is 18 °C (64 °F) and annual rainfall is 2739 mm. The state is situated in the Eastern Himalayas and it shares its border with countries like Tibet, Nepal and Bhutan. Mt Kanchendzonga (8585m) which is the third highest peak in the world is situated at Sikkim. According to 2011 census, population of state was 610,577 with male population of 323,070 and female population of 287,507. The literacy rate in the state is 81.40 percent. The density of the state is 86 people per $km^2$ (Census,2011). The cattle population in the state was 264,860 in number (BAHS,2019). The state has four district- East, West, North, and South (Registrar General of India, 1989).

### 3.1.1 Description of the study area

**Table 3.1.1.** Dairy Development Status in Sikkim

| Sl. No. | Parameter | Quantity |
|---|---|---|
| 1. | Milk Production 2017-18 (000 tonnes) | 58.67 |
| 2. | Per Capita Availability -2017-18 (grams/day) | 244 |
| 3. | No. of Milk Potential Villages<br>(% of total no. of villages) | 300<br>(66.52%) |
| 5. | Number of organized Dairy Cooperative Societies (DCS) | 497 |
| 6. | Number of farmers enrolled under DCS | 13687 |
| 7. | Average milk procurement by DCS (in TKgPD)<br>(% of milk production) | 36<br>(22.40) |

(*Source:* State Dairy Profiles, 2019, DAHD&F)

The table 3.1.1, gives a detailed information about the milk production in the state. The average milk procured by DCS in the state was 22.40 percent. Per capita availability of milk production was 244gms/day.

**Table 3.1.2.** Livestock population in Sikkim

| Sl. No. | Livestock | Quantity (000) |
|---|---|---|
| 1. | Indigenous Cattle | 148.010 |
| 2. | Crossbred Cattle | 116.850 |
| 3. | Goat | 90.506 |
| 4. | Pig | 27.32 |
| 5. | Yak | 5.219 |
| 6. | Sheep | 0.816 |
| 7. | Buffalo | 1.144 |
| 8. | Poultry | 580.864 |

(*Source:* 20th Livestock Census,2019)

The table 3.1.2, provides information about livestock population in the state. The number of indigenous cattle was more than crossbred cattle in the state.

**Table 3.1.3.** Status of milk production by Exotic and Indigenous Cattle in Sikkim

| Sl. No. | Parameters | Exotic/Crossbred | Indigenous |
|---|---|---|---|
| 1. | Estimate of Milk Production (000' tones) | 60.85 | 0 |
| 2. | No. of Animal In-Milk (000 nos.) | 32.21 | 0 |
| 3. | Average Yield Per In- Milk Animal (Kg/ha) | 5.18 | 0 |

(*Source:* Basic Animal Husbandry Statistics, 2019)

The table 3.1.3, shows information about the milk production by the exotic/ crossbred and indigenous cattle in the state. The table indicates that the exotic/ crossbred cow are performing well in milk production of the state.

**Table 3.1.4.** Breed-wise cattle population in Sikkim

| Sl. No. | Breed | Total nos. |
|---|---|---|
| 1. | Crossbred Jersey | 125,247 |
| 2. | Siri | 11,254 |
| 3. | Non-Descriptive | 2694 |
| 4. | Crossbred Holstein Fries | 1100 |
| 5. | Jersey | 122 |
| 6. | Holstein Fries | 50 |

(*Source:* District-wise Breed- wise Cattle Population, 2013, DAHD&F)

The table 3.1.4, shows the breed wise population in the state. The state has highest number of crossbred jerseys, followed by siri cattle.

**Table 3.1.5.** Status of crop cultivation in Sikkim

| Sl. No. | Crop | Area (000'ha) | Production (000'tones) | Productivity (Kg/ha) |
|---|---|---|---|---|
| 1. | Rice | 9.50 | 17.64 | 1856.24 |
| 2. | Wheat | 0.17 | 0.19 | 1079.26 |
| 3. | Maize | 38.46 | 67.97 | 1769.34 |
| 4. | Finger Millet | 2.47 | 2.55 | 1031.65 |
| 5. | Barley | 0.42 | 0.45 | 1072.64 |
| 6. | Buckwheat | 3.43 | 3.35 | 976.24 |
| 7. | Pulses | 5.35 | 5.10 | 954.21 |
| 8. | Oilseeds | 6.28 | 5.80 | 924.55 |

(*Source:* ENVIS Sikkim: Status of Environment and Related Issues, Agriculture, 2017-18)

The table 3.1.5, provides information about various crop cultivation in the state. Maize is one of the important cereal crops grown in Sikkim. It is cultivated in area of around 38.46 hectare, which is about 35-40% cultivable land. Oilseed crops like mustard is grown for oil extraction and fodder purpose. Other fodder crops like buckwheat, finger millet and barley are also cultivated in the state.

### 3.1.2 Selection of the state

Firstly, Sikkim is the only 100 percent organic state in the country. Sikkim was declared organic state by honourable Prime Minister on January 18, 2016. The state is rich in biodiversity. Agriculture and animal husbandry is an integral part of the rural population in the state. The state has a strong base of livestock based rural livelihoods. Eighty percent of the rural population owns livestock and 70 percent of the main work force was contributed through it (Sikkim Livestock Policy,2011). The contribution of livestock to the state economy is 6 percent to 7 percent of NSDP (DAHLFVS, GOS, 2021). The employment through the livestock sector is 4.5 percent per annum. Nearly, 85 percent of the species and livestock are owned by small and marginal farmers of the state. (Sikkim Livestock Policy,2011). Total asset value of the livestock is estimated to be more than Rs.995.27 million, out of which 46 percent is from milk. The livestock impact on rural income of Sikkim is found to be 14.32 percent from milk and 0.5 to 3.2 percent from other livestock, (Sikkim Livestock Policy,2011). Around 60 percent of the income in rural household is contributed through livestock farming. Keeping that information in view the current study has been conducted in the state of Sikkim.

### 3.1.3 Selection of East district

East district is one of the administrative districts of Sikkim. It covers an area of 964 km sq. It lies between 27 °19' N and 88 °36' E. It is situated in the south-east corner of the state. According to Census (2011), East district had a population of 2,81,293, in which 1,50,260 were male and 1,31,033 were female. It was confirmed as most populated district with 46.29 percent of the total population of the state and the rural population of 1,60,543. Gangtok is located in East Sikkim which is the capital of the state. Literacy rate in this district is 79.99 percent (2011, Census). The major crops grown in the district are, rice, maize, finger millet, soya bean and mustard.

The specific reason for selection of East district is given in the following paragraphs:

- The cattle population was highest in number in East district compared to other three districts.

**Table 3.1.6.** Cattle populations in the state of Sikkim

| District | No. of cattle population |
|---|---|
| East | 46826 |
| West | 14011 |
| North | 37179 |
| South | 42451 |

(*Source:* District-wise Breed- wise Cattle Population, 2013, DAHD&F)

- One of the apex cooperative body, Sikkim Cooperative Milk Producer Union Ltd (SCMPUL) formed in the year 1980, is located in East district of Sikkim. The Sikkim milk union is the largest cooperative of milk in the state. There were 405 number of milk collection centers under the milk union. (Livestock Sector towards Rural Prosperity, 2016)

- Under the SCMPUL, two milk processing plants one at Tadong, Gangtok (East district) and other at Karfectar, Jorthang (South district) with processing capacity of 10,000 and 5000 liter per day were present.
- The number of households owning livestock was 2nd highest in East district of Sikkim.
- The researcher was well acquainted with the culture, socio custom and language of the study area which enabled the researcher in building a good rapport with the respondent and getting reliable information.

## 3.2 Sampling Plan

The study has been conducted in Sikkim. East district has been selected purposively for the research.

**3.2.1 Selection of block:** From the East district four blocks have been selected randomly. Blocks namely Khamdong, Nandok, Rakdong Tintek and Ranka were selected.

**3.2.2 Selection of Village:** Five villages under each block were selected randomly. From each village 10 women farmers were selected. The total respondent was 200 in number. The respondents were selected under the criteria that the farmer should own at least one dairy animal. The list of the villages selected for the study are presented below.

**Table 3.2.** List of randomly selected village

| Sl. No. | Name of the block | Name of the Village | Number of respondents |
|---|---|---|---|
| 1. | Nandok | Merrung | 10 |
| | | Chongay | 10 |
| | | Maney Dara | 10 |
| | | Dothapu | 10 |
| | | Kopi Bari | 10 |
| 2. | Ranka | Rai Goan | 10 |
| | | Sama Sevik | 10 |
| | | Upper Lingdum | 10 |
| | | Rey Mendu | 10 |
| | | Tephyak Mendu | 10 |
| 3. | Rakdong Tintek | Upper Rakdong | 10 |
| | | Lower Rakdong | 10 |
| | | Dara Gaon | 10 |
| | | Chuba | 10 |
| | | Rakshay | 10 |

| 4. | Khamdong | Ramitay | 10 |
|---|---|---|---|
| | | Aritar | 10 |
| | | Dung Dung | 10 |
| | | Budang | 10 |
| | | Lingzey | 10 |

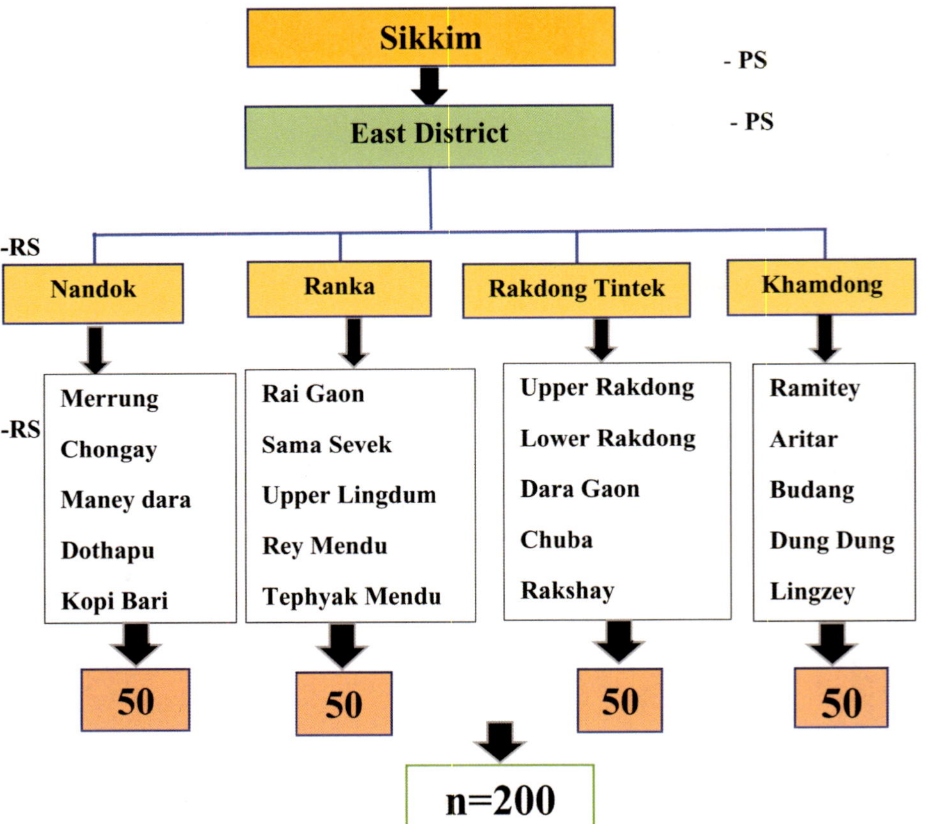


**PS -Purposive sampling, RS- Random sampling**

**Fig. 1.** Sampling plan

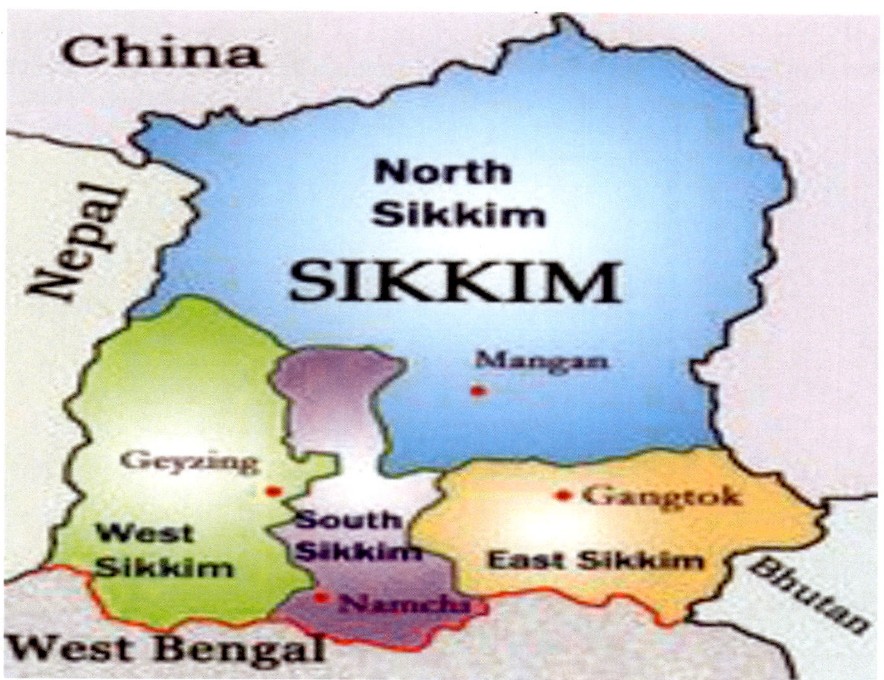


**Map 1.** Map of Sikkim showing districts
(*Source:* www.mapsofindia.com)

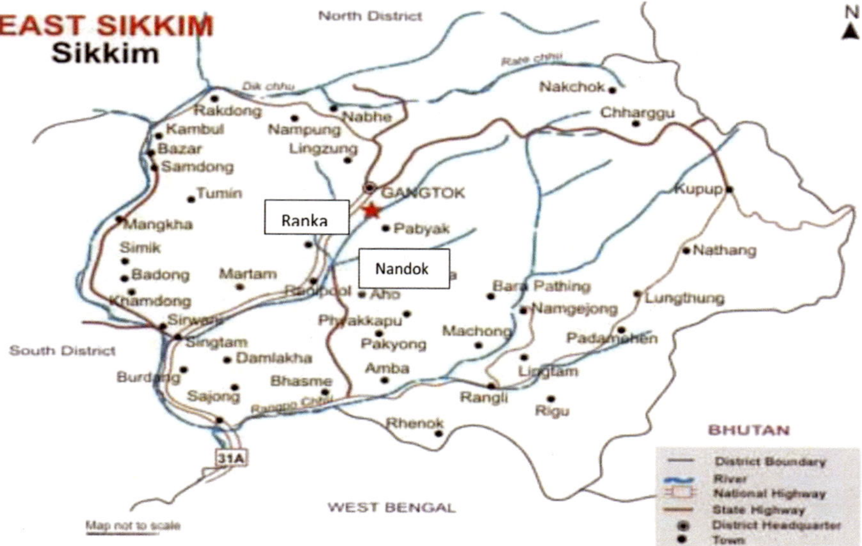


**Map 2.** Map of Sikkim showing blocks
(*Source:* www.mapsofindia.com)

## 3.3 Measurement of variables

The following variables were selected under the study. The detailed measurement procedure of the variables is given in the following paragraphs.

**Table 3.3.** Variables and their measurement

<table>
<tr><th>Sl. No.</th><th>Variable</th><th>Measurement</th></tr>
<tr><td>1.</td><td>Age</td><td rowspan="4">Schedule was developed</td></tr>
<tr><td>2.</td><td>Education</td></tr>
<tr><td>3.</td><td>Marital status</td></tr>
<tr><td>4.</td><td>Family size</td></tr>
<tr><td>5.</td><td>Family type</td><td rowspan="6">Schedule was developed</td></tr>
<tr><td>6.</td><td>Milk production per day (in liters)</td></tr>
<tr><td>7.</td><td>Social status</td></tr>
<tr><td>8.</td><td>Farming experience in dairying (in years)</td></tr>
<tr><td>9.</td><td>Land holding</td></tr>
<tr><td>10.</td><td>Herd size</td></tr>
<tr><td>11.</td><td>Annual Income through dairying (in Rs)</td><td rowspan="5">Schedule was developed</td></tr>
<tr><td>12.</td><td>Livestock possession</td></tr>
<tr><td>13.</td><td>Source of information</td></tr>
<tr><td>14.</td><td>Occupation</td></tr>
<tr><td>15.</td><td>Asset possession</td></tr>
<tr><td>16.</td><td>Access to finance</td><td rowspan="3">Schedule was developed</td></tr>
<tr><td>17.</td><td>Social participation</td></tr>
<tr><td>18.</td><td>Time utilization pattern</td></tr>
<tr><td>19.</td><td>Role of women in dairying.</td><td>Schedule was developed</td></tr>
<tr><td>20.</td><td>Socio-economic empowerment of farm women in dairying.</td><td>Index was developed</td></tr>
</table>

## 3.4 Operationalization of definition

**3.4.1** Age refers to the chronological age of the respondent at the time of data collection. The age of farm women was classified as follows:

| Sl. No. | Category | Years |
|---|---|---|
| 1. | Young | Up to 35 |
| 2. | Middle | 36 to 50 |
| 3. | Old | Above 50 |

**3.4.2 Education** refers to the total number of years of formal schooling the respondent had received. Education of the respondent was denoted by following scoring pattern:

| Sl. No. | Category | Score |
|---|---|---|
| 1. | Illiterate | 0 |
| 2. | Primary School | 1 |
| 3. | Middle School (up to class 10) | 2 |
| 4. | Higher Secondary School | 3 |
| 5. | Graduate and above | 4 |

**3.4.3 Marital** status refers to decision that shows an individual's relation with their partners. The following scoring pattern was followed:

| Sl. No. | Category | Scores |
|---|---|---|
| 1. | Married | 1 |
| 2. | Unmarried | 2 |
| 3. | Widow | 3 |

**3.4.4 Family size** refers to the number of family member living together in a single household. Family size has been categorized according to the following pattern:

| Sl. No. | Category | Numbers | Scores |
|---|---|---|---|
| 1. | Small | Up to 4 | 1 |
| 2. | Large | Above 4 | 2 |

**3.4.5 Family type** represents the different form of family the respondents are having. It can be either nuclear or joint family. It has been denoted by the following scoring pattern:

| Sl. No. | Type | Scores |
|---|---|---|
| 1. | Nuclear | 1 |
| 2. | Joint | 2 |

**3.4.6 Milk production per day** refers to the total amount of milk produced by the dairy cattle on the day before interview. It has been categorized into the following categories by using cumulative square root frequency method:

| Sl. No. | Category | Milk production (in Liters) |
|---|---|---|
| 1. | Low | <7 |
| 2. | Medium | 7-13.50 |
| 3. | High | >13.50 |

**3.4.7 Social status** refers to group of individuals whose privilege and obligation are inherited by birth. The variables were measured with the help of caste system prevailing in the society. The following scoring pattern was followed:

| Sl. No. | Category | Scores |
|---|---|---|
| 1. | General | 1 |
| 2. | Other Backward Caste (OBC) | 2 |
| 3. | Scheduled Caste (SC) | 3 |
| 4. | Scheduled Tribe (ST) | 4 |

**3.4.8 Farming experience** in dairying refers to the involvement of the farm women in dairy farming in a completed year at the time of interview. It has been categorized into following categories using cumulative square root frequency method:

| Sl. No. | Category | Farming experience (in years) |
|---|---|---|
| 1. | Low | < 13.08 years |
| 2. | Medium | 13.08-28.40 years |
| 3. | High | >28.40 years |

**3.4.9 Land holding** refers to the total area of land in acres or hectare, under the possession of respondent at the time of data collection. The land holding has been categorized into the following groups using cumulative square root frequency method:

| Sl. No. | Category | Land holdings |
|---|---|---|
| 1. | Marginal | < 1 ha |
| 2. | Small | 1 to 2 ha |

**3.4.10 Herd size** refers to the total number of animals in the herd possessed by the respondent at the time of investigation. It has been categorized into the following categories by using cumulative square root frequency method:

| Sl. No. | Category | Herd size |
|---|---|---|
| 1. | Small | <3 |
| 2. | Medium | 3-5 |
| 3. | Large | >5 |

**3.4.11 Annual income through dairying** refers to the amount of money earned by the respondent in one fiscal year through dairying. It has been categorized into low, medium and high category by using cumulative square root frequency method:

| Sl. No. | Category | Annual income (in Rs) |
|---|---|---|
| 1. | Low | <0.99 lakhs |
| 2. | Medium | 0.99-4.19 lakhs |
| 3. | High | >4.19 lakhs |

**3.4.12 Livestock possession** refers to the total number of livestock owned by the respondent during the time of investigation. It has been categorized into low, medium and high category by using cumulative square root frequency method:

| Sl. No. | Category | Livestock possession |
|---|---|---|
| 1. | Small | <7 |
| 2. | Medium | 7-15 |
| 3. | Large | >15 |

**3.4.13 Source of information** refers to any source through which the farm women get information about the dairying and other farm related activities. It has been categorized into low, medium and high category by using cumulative square root frequency method:

| Sl. No. | Category | Source of information |
|---|---|---|
| 1. | Low | <9 |
| 2. | Medium | 9-14 |
| 3. | High | >14 |

**3.4.14 Occupation** refers to the work carried out by the respondent through the farming enterprise, which generate income in their household. The scoring patten used were as follows:

| Sl. No. | Category | Scores |
|---|---|---|
| 1. | Dairy farmer | 1 |
| 2. | Agri+ Dairy farmer | 2 |
| 3. | Labor work + Agri+ Dairy farmer | 3 |
| 4. | Government service+ Dairy farming | 4 |

**3.4.15 Asset possession** refers to the materials possessed by the respondents in their farm. Materials like land possession, machineries, insurance, buildings etc. which indicates their standard of living for which the response recorded was either "yes" or "no" based on their asset possession.

**3.4.16 Access to finance** refers to the degree to which respondent take credit from any formal institution or non-formal institution, like banks, friends, self-help group, village head etc. The response recorded was either "yes" or "no" based on their access to finance.

**3.4.17 Social participation** refers to degree of involvement of the farm women in an organization or social group, like gram panchayat, cooperative society, self-help group, anganwadi groups and religious group etc. The response recorded was either "yes" or "no" based on their participation.

**3.4.18 Time utilization pattern** refers to the degree of utilization of time in a certain pattern by the farm women on various activities in their farm in a day. Activities like collection of fodder, preparation of feed and fodder, cleaning of feed and fodder, milking of cattle, selling of milk was taken into consideration. All the activities were categorized into low, medium and high using cumulative square frequency method.

### 3.4.19 Differential role accomplished by women dairy farmer with respect to their social strata

It operationalized various dairy related activities performed by the respondent. The activities were divided into breeding aspect, feeding aspect, marketing aspect, health care aspect, housing aspect, economic aspect and decision-making aspect. Basically, two variables had been taken into consideration in view of social strata for measuring the differential role. They were caste of the respondent and annual income through dairying. The response category for each statement under different aspect were regularly, often, sometimes, and never. The scores given were 4,3,2,1 respectively. For this cross tabulation was carried out for the various dairy related activities under each aspect with respect to caste and annual income of the women dairy farmers and frequency and percentage were taken into consideration.

### 3.4.20 Socio-economic empowerment

It operationalizes the process in which the farm women gain control over their own lives and assets by becoming self-confident and making important decision in changing the society into better place to live in. Index was developed for the socio-economic empowerment.

For measuring the socio-economic empowerment index (SEI) five dimensions of empowerment were selected. They were:

### 'Social' Dimension

Social dimension in empowerment refers to the development in which women acquire a societal identification in the community, a sense of communal belonging in the society, where she become self-confident and self -reliant to make her own decision independently.

### 'Economic' Dimension

Economic dimension in empowerment refers to the process, where the women take authority over the financial matter from the household level to professional level. It leads women to attain liberty to live their life as per their choice.

### 'Freedom to Mobility'- Dimension

Freedom to mobility dimension in empowerment refers to independence in the movement of women to various places without any restriction, which will help them to gain awareness about the various opportunities for their self-development.

### 'Technical Knowledge Possession'- Dimension

Technical knowledge possession dimension in empowerment refers to the process in which the women acquire technical know how about new innovation and technology in a particular field, which will lead them to establish their own enterprise and become self- sustainable through the gain of technological knowledge.

### 'Decision making factor'- Dimension

Decision making factor in empowerment is an important aspect for determining the worth of women in general. It refers to the power possessed by the women to take important decision, from domestic affairs to their professional life, without any hinderance.

For development of the index, items/statements along with dimensions were sent for judges rating. Scientist, subject matter specialist, assistant professor and expert in the field of women empowerment were selected as judges. They were requested to allot appropriate weightage to the five dimensions, out of 100. Under each dimension statements were provided with 3-point continuum i.e. "Most relevant", "Relevant" and "Irrelevant" for which scores provided were 3, 2, 1. The statements were also sent to the same judges by using google form format via email to suggest the degree of relevancy of statements. Out of 150 judges about 58 responses were received and the means of the dimensions were calculated and weightage was taken. The relevancy weightage (RW)was calculated by using the given formula and the statement having more than 0.7 relevancy value were selected for index preparation. Total of 44 statements were taken in consideration under the five dimensions of empowerment

$$RW = \frac{\textbf{Most relevant responses} * 3 + \textbf{Relevant responses} * 2 + \textbf{Not relevant responses} * 1}{\textbf{Maximum possible scores}}$$

**Table 3.4.** Weightage given to the five dimensions of empowerment according to judges

| Weightage to dimensions | Scores (out of 100) |
|---|---|
| (W1) Social dimension (SD) | 19.67 |
| (W2) Economic dimension (ED) | 23.05 |
| (W3) Freedom to mobility dimension (FMD) | 24.57 |
| (W4) Technical knowledge dimension (TKD) | 16.06 |
| (W4) Decision making dimension (DMD) | 16.65 |

The table 3.4 is showing the weightage of the different dimensions of empowerment according to judges. According to judges, freedom to mobility and economic dimension got the highest and second highest weightage.

### 3.4.20.1 Weighted scores

Weighted score for each dimension was calculated by multiplying the percentage scores of each dimension by their respective weights. It was done as (W1xSD), (W2xED), (W3xFMD), (W4xTKD) and (W5xDMD)

### 3.4.20.2 Socio-economic Empowerment Index (SEI)

It was obtained by adding the weighted score of each of the dimension of a respondent and then divided by 100. The formula is given as follows:

$$\mathrm{SEI} = \frac{(\mathrm{W1} \times \mathrm{SD}) + (\mathrm{W2} \times \mathrm{ED}) + (\mathrm{W3} \times \mathrm{FMD}) + (\mathrm{W4} \times \mathrm{TKD}) + (\mathrm{W5} \times \mathrm{DMD})}{100}$$

The categorization of the respondent on the basis of empowerment scores was done as follows, by using cumulative square root method:

| Sl. No. | Categories | Empowerment score | Score |
|---|---|---|---|
| 1. | Low | <59.74 | 1 |
| 2. | Medium | 59.74-80.74 | 2 |
| 3. | High | >80.74 | 3 |

Chi square and ANOVA, Post hoc test was carried to measure the degree of association among various socio-economic variables with the empowerment scores.

### 3.4.21 Feedback given by the respondent related to dairy farming

Feedback have been operationalized as the response of hindrance faced by the respondents who were practicing dairy farming in the study area. The feedbacks were presented to the respondents, which were classified according to economical aspects, technical aspects, administrative aspects, information networking aspects, independence in decision making aspects, respectively.

The respondents were asked to rank the statements given under each aspect according to the degree of importance as conceived by them. For measuring the ranks Garrett's ranking technique was applied.

### Garrett's ranking technique

This method was used for finding out the significant factor which influences the reaction of respondents. According to this method, respondents have to assign rank for all factors and the result of such ranking has been converted into score value by using the given formula:

$$\text{Percent Position} = \frac{100(R_{ij} - 0.5)}{Nj}$$

Where;

Rij= Rank given for the ith factor by jth respondents

Nj= Number of factor ranked by jth respondents

### 3.5 Method of data collection

A structured interview schedule was prepared for the data collection. Necessary care was taken to verify that the question formulated were clear, specific, complete, unambiguous and comprehensive. The primary data was collected from the respondent mostly through personal interview so to build a good rapport and to obtain valid information.

### 3.6 Statistical tools used

The statistical tools used for the study were mean, standard deviation, standard error of mean etc.

#### 3.6.1 Frequency

It determines number of respondents in the cell.

#### 3.6.2 Percentage

It is calculated by dividing the frequency value by the total number of respondents multiplied by 100.

#### 3.6.3 Mean

It is the summation of scores divided by the total number of respondents present.

The formula for mean is as follows:

$$\text{Mean} = \frac{\sum_{i=1}^{n} xi}{n} \{i = 1, 2, 3, .....n\}$$

Where,

X= mean

$\sum Xi$ = Sum of scores

n = no. of respondents

### 3.6.4 Standard Error of the Mean

Standard Error of the Mean is defined as the standard deviation of the sampling distribution of mean. The formula for the standard deviation of error of the mean is as follows:

$$\sigma M = \frac{\sigma}{\sqrt{N}}$$

Apart from that Chi square test and Analysis of Variance (ANOVA) test was used to draw meaningful conclusion of the study. SPSS 23.0 statistical package was used to analyze the data.

# 4

# Results and Disscussion

This chapter presents the analysis, interpretation and discussion of the collected data from the study area in an effort to attain the objective of the study. The data collected were analyzed with appropriate statistical test and presented in a systematic format.

The results of the study are presented under the following subheadings:

## 4.1 Distribution of respondents according to different socio-economic variables

Basic information of the respondents under the study has been given according to the socio-economic characteristic of the respondents. Variables like age, education, marital status, family size, family type, milk production per day, social status, farming experience, herd size, land holding and annual income are presented in the following table 4.1

**Table 4.1.** Distribution of respondents according to socio-economic variables with respect to frequency and percentage

**(n=200)**

| Sl. No. | Variables | Categories | Frequency | Percentage (%) |
|---|---|---|---|---|
| 1. | Age | Young (up to 35) | 54 | 27.00 |
| | | Middle (36-50) | 76 | 38.00 |
| | | Old (>50) | 70 | 35.00 |
| 2. | Education | Illiterate (0) | 55 | 27.50 |
| | | Primary (1) | 58 | 29.00 |
| | | Secondary (2) | 42 | 21.00 |
| | | Higher sec. (3) | 24 | 12.00 |
| | | Graduate and above (4) | 21 | 10.50 |
| 3. | Marital status | Married (1) | 179 | 89.50 |
| | | Unmarried (2) | 15 | 7.50 |
| | | Widow (3) | 6 | 3.00 |
| 4. | Family type | Nuclear (0) | 134 | 67.00 |
| | | Joint (1) | 66 | 33.00 |

| Sl. No. | Variables | Categories | Frequency | Percentage (%) |
|---|---|---|---|---|
| 5. | Family Size | Small Family (up to 4) | 79 | 39.50 |
| | | Large Family (>4) | 121 | 60.50 |
| 6. | Milk production/day (in litres) | Low (<7lit) | 131 | 65.50 |
| | | Medium (7-13.50 lit) | 50 | 25.00 |
| | | High (>13.50lit) | 19 | 9.50 |
| 7. | Social status | General | 90 | 45.00 |
| | | OBC | 19 | 9.50 |
| | | SC | 24 | 12.00 |
| | | ST | 67 | 33.50 |
| 8. | Farming Experience in dairying (In years) | Low (<13.08) | 86 | 43.00 |
| | | Medium (13.08-28.40) | 51 | 25.50 |
| | | High (>28.40) | 63 | 31.50 |
| 9. | Landholding | Marginal (<1ha) | 190 | 95.00 |
| | | Small (1-2ha) | 10 | 5.00 |
| 10. | Herd Size | Small (<3) | 126 | 63.00 |
| | | Medium (3-5) | 54 | 27.00 |
| | | Large (>5) | 20 | 10.00 |
| 11. | Annual income through dairying (in Rs) | Low (<0.99 lakhs) | 117 | 58.50 |
| | | Medium (0.99-4.19 lakhs) | 76 | 38.00 |
| | | High (>4.19 lakhs) | 7 | 3.50 |
| 12. | Livestock possession | Small (<7) | 96 | 48.00 |
| | | Medium (7-15) | 91 | 45.50 |
| | | Large (>15) | 13 | 6.50 |
| 13. | Source of information | Low (<9) | 59 | 29.50 |
| | | Medium (9-14) | 84 | 42.00 |
| | | High (>14) | 57 | 28.50 |
| 14. | Occupation | Dairy farming | 115 | 57.50 |
| | | Agri+ Dairy farming | 28 | 14.00 |
| | | Labour work + Agri+ Dairy farming | 44 | 22.00 |
| | | Govt service+ Dairy farming | 13 | 6.50 |

### 4.1.1 Age

From the table 4.1, it can be inferred that, 38.00 percent of the respondents were middle aged, 35.00 percent were old aged while, 27.00 percent of the respondents were young aged. This shows that maximum respondents belonged to middle and old age group as they perceived dairying as a gainful venture, while the young age group were reluctant to take dairy farming as a profession due to technological advancement in other fields. Fig. 2 shows categories of age of respondents. The above results are in support with the finding of Gupta *et al.* (2020), Khan *et al.* (2014) and Rathod *et al.* (2011).

### 4.1.2 Education

From the table 4.1, it was revealed that, 27.50 percent of the respondents were illiterate, while 29.00 percent of the respondents were having primary education. On the other hand, 43.50 percent of the respondents were having secondary, higher and graduate level of education, thus it can be said that highly educated people were less engaged in dairy farming as compared to the illiterate and primary educated group because they were having wider job opportunity. Fig. 3 shows education level of respondents. Similar results have been found in study of Kaur (2015) and Dash *et al.* (2020)

### 4.1.3Marital status

The table 4.1, reported that, majority of the respondents (89.50%) were married. This proved that married women were more engaged in dairy activities compared to unmarried and widow women. The reason for this can be due to the mutual responsibility shared by the husband and wife for cattle rearing, making their work easier. These results are in support with the study of Rathod *et al.* (2011), Yadav and Revanna (2017), Dash *et al.* (2020)

### 4.1.4 Family type

The table 4.1 conveyed that, majority of the respondents (67.00%) belonged to the nuclear family and 33.00 percent belonged to joint family. The reason behind this is that, the women belonging to the nuclear family have more time to devote in dairy farming activities as they have lesser member in the family to take care of, than the women belonging to the joint family. The results are in line with the study of Yadav and Revanna (2017), Gupta *et al.* (2020)

### 4.1.5 Family size

From the table 4.1, the result revealed that majority of the respondents (60.50%) belonged to large family (>4 member) while 39.50 percent belonged to small family size (up to 4).

### 4.1.6 Milk production per day (in litres)

From the table 4.1, it was found that majority of the respondents (65.50%) belonged to low milk production category, 25.00 percent belonged to medium milk production category and 9.50 percent belonged to high milk production category. The reason for this is that most of the respondents practiced subsistence dairy farming and were usually keeping local breeds which produced on an average 5-liter milk per day. Fig. 5 shows milk production per day. The results are in line with the study of Kaur *et al.* (2019)

### 4.1.7 Social status

From the table 4.1, it can be seen that 45.00 percent of the respondents belonged to General category followed by 33.50 percent belonged to Scheduled Tribe, while 12.00 percent belonged to Scheduled Caste and 9.50 per cent belonged to Other Backward Caste. These results are in support with the finding of Devi (2016), Kaur *et al.* (2019) and Gupta *et al.* (2020), where they found that maximum respondents practicing dairying belonged to General category.

### 4.1.8 Farming experience in dairying (in years)

From the table 4.1, it can be inferred that 43.00 percent of the respondents had low experience in dairy farming, while only 31.50 percent of the respondent had high experience in dairy farming.

### 4.1.9 Land holding

From the table 4.1, the result exhibited that majority of the respondents (95.00%) belonged to marginal land holding, whereas 5.00 percent belonged to small land holding. Similar results were observed by Kathiriya *et al.* (2013), Yadav and Revanna (2017)

### 4.1.10 Herd size

From the table 4.1, it can be said that 63.00 percent respondents had small herd size, followed by 27.00 percent had medium herd size and 10.00 percent had large herd size. The reason for majority having small herd size might be due to lack of surplus land for rearing cattle, cultivating fodder and non-availability of green fodder during the winter season. Similar findings were observed by Nithya and Selvaraj (2018) and Kaur *et al.* (2019)

### 4.1.11 Annual income through dairying (in Rs)

The perusal of the table 4.1, revealed that 58.50 percent respondents belonged to low annual income group, followed by 38.00 percent belonged to medium and 3.50 percent belonged to high income group. Similar results were seen in findings of Kathiriya *et al.* (2013) and Kaur (2015)

### 4.1.12 Livestock possession

From the table 4.1, it was found that 48.00 percent of the respondents had small livestock possession, while 45.50 percent had medium livestock possession. On the other hand, only 6.50 percent respondents fell in large livestock possession category.

### 4.1.13 Source of information

From the table 4.1, it can be said that 42.00 percent of respondents under medium category had highest source of information related to dairy and other farm activities as compared to 29.50 percent respondents fell under low category and 28.50 percent respondents fell under high category.

### 4.1.14 Occupation

From the table 4.1, it can be said that majority (57.50%) of the respondents were dairy farmers by profession, while 22.00 percent worked as labor and used to do agriculture and dairy farming, 14.00 percent respondents practiced agriculture as well as dairy farming and 6.50 percent were government employed. Fig. 12 represents bar diagram of occupation of the respondents.

### 4.1.15 Asset possession

**Table 4.2.** Distribution of respondents according to their asset possession

| Sl. No. | Categories | Yes | % | No | % |
|---|---|---|---|---|---|
| 1. | Land possession | 2 | 1.00 | 198 | 99.00 |
| 2. | Buildings | 103 | 51.50 | 97 | 48.50 |
| 3. | Farm machineries | 32 | 16.00 | 168 | 84.00 |
| 4. | Insurance | 82 | 41.00 | 118 | 59.00 |
| 5. | Others | 97 | 48.50 | 103 | 51.50 |

From the table 4.2, the study revealed that majority (51.50%) of the respondents possessed building, while 41.00 percent possessed insurance in their name and only 1.00 percent had land possession.

### 4.1.16 Access to finance

**Table 4.3.** Distribution of respondents according to their access to finance

| Sl. No. | Categories | Yes | % | No | % |
|---|---|---|---|---|---|
| 1. | Bank | 81 | 40.50 | 119 | 59.50 |
| 2. | Friends | 135 | 67.50 | 65 | 32.50 |
| 3. | Self Help Group | 79 | 39.50 | 121 | 60.50 |
| 4. | Village head | 0 | 0 | 0 | 0 |

From the table 4.3, the study exposed that 67.50 percent respondents were taking loan from informal source like friends. On the other hand, 40.50 percent of the respondents were taking loan from bank and 39.50 percent were having access to finance through self-help group.

### 4.1.17 Social participation

**Table 4.4.** Distribution of respondents according to their social participation

| Sl. No. | Categories | Participation | % | Non- participation | % |
|---|---|---|---|---|---|
| 1. | Gram panchayat | 164 | 82.00 | 36 | 18.00 |
| 2. | Cooperative society | 126 | 63.00 | 74 | 37.00 |
| 3. | Self Help Group | 129 | 64.50 | 71 | 35.50 |
| 4. | Anganwadi | 51 | 25.50 | 149 | 74.50 |
| 5. | Religious group | 199 | 99.50 | 1 | 0.50 |

From the table 4.4, the study exhibited that majority (82.00%) of the respondents participated in gram panchayat meetings, 63.00 percent of the respondents participated in cooperative society. On the other hand, 64.50 percent of the respondents participated in self-help group and 99.50 percent participated in religious group.

### 4.1.18 Time utilization pattern

**Table 4.5.** Distribution of respondents according to their time utilization pattern

| Sl. No. | Activities | Category (mins/day) | Frequency | Percentage |
|---|---|---|---|---|
| 1. | Collection of fodder | Low (<87.70) | 69 | 34.50 |
| | | Medium (87.70-171.40) | 63 | 31.50 |
| | | High (>171.40) | 68 | 34.00 |
| 2. | Preparation of feed and feeding | Low (<46.70) | 82 | 41.00 |
| | | Medium (46.70-72.20) | 89 | 44.50 |
| | | High (>72.20) | 29 | 14.50 |
| 3. | Cleaning of animal and cow shed | Low (<31.30) | 85 | 42.50 |
| | | Medium (31.30-57.50) | 37 | 18.50 |
| | | High (>57.50) | 78 | 39.00 |
| 4. | Milking of cattle | Low (<15.80) | 80 | 40.00 |
| | | Medium (15.80-24.40) | 45 | 22.50 |
| | | High (>24.40) | 75 | 37.50 |
| 5. | Selling of milk | Low (<36.60) | 86 | 43.00 |
| | | Medium (36.6-89.00) | 71 | 35.50 |
| | | High (<89.00) | 43 | 21.50 |

From the table 4.5, it can be seen that under the time utilization pattern, activities like collection of fodder, preparation of feed and feeding, cleaning of animal and cow shed, milking of cattle and selling of milk were taken into consideration along with the amount of time they take in performing these activities in a day.The study revealed that in the case of "collection of fodder" 34.50 percent of the respondent were taking less than one hour and twenty minutes in undertaking the activity, while 34.00 percent were taking more than 2 hours in undertaking the said activity because of lack of availability of fodder in the nearby area and hence the respondents had to go to forest to collect the fodder. For "preparation of feed and feeding" nearly half of the total respondent (44.50%) was taking medium time between an hour or more. In the case of "cleaning of animal and cow shed", 42.50 percent of the respondent were taking less time i.e., about 30 minutes in undertaking the activity, while 39.00 percent were taking high time nearly an hour in performing the activity. Regarding "milking of cattle" 40.00 percent respondent were taking less time (about 15 minutes) in milking of cattle, while 37.50 percent respondent were taking high time (about more than 20 minutes) in milking cattle. For selling of milk 43.00 percent of the respondent under low category were taking less than 36 minutes in selling of milk.

## 4.2 Assessing the differential role accomplished by women dairy farmers from different social strata in the study area

The present study has made an attempt to measure the differential role accomplished by the respondents in the study area with respect to their social strata. In the current study mainly two variables i.e., caste of the respondent and annual income acquired through dairying by the respondent have been taken into consideration. The result of the objective is given in the following paragraphs:

### 4.2.1. Distribution of respondents for differential role accomplished by women dairy farmer with respect to social caste

In the study area, four major social caste were prevailing. They were General category, Other Backward Caste (OBC), Scheduled Caste (SC) and Scheduled Tribe (ST). According to these caste categories differential roles accomplished by the respondents were analyzed. The differential roles were categorized under breeding, feeding, marketing, health care, housing, economic and decision-making aspects

**Distribution of respondents according to socio-economic variables with respect to percentage (n=200)**

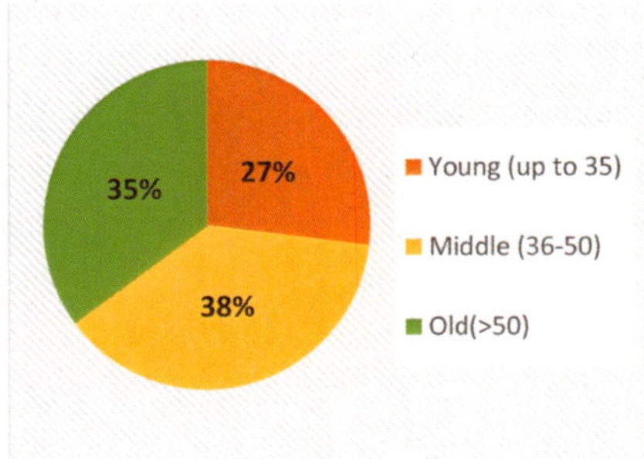


**Fig. 2.** Age

| | Percentage |
|---|---|
| Graduate and above | 10.5 |
| Higher sec. | 12 |
| Secondary | 21 |
| Primary | 29 |
| Illiterate | 27.5 |

**Fig. 3.** Education

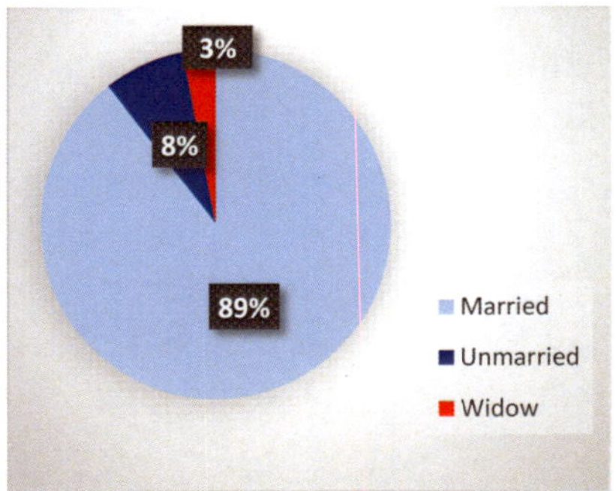


**Fig. 4.** Marital Status

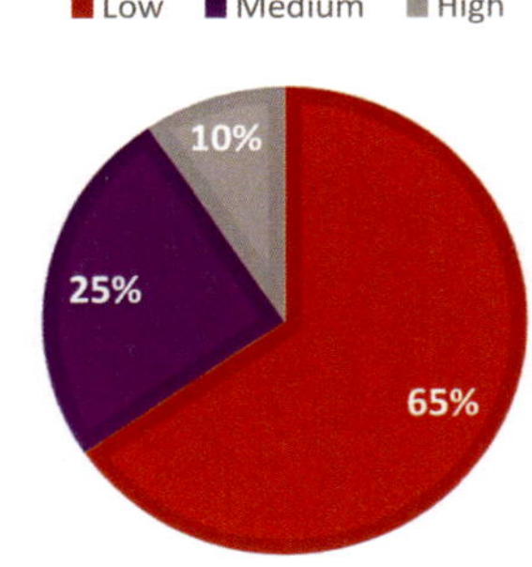


**Fig. 5.** Milk Production/ Day (In Litres)

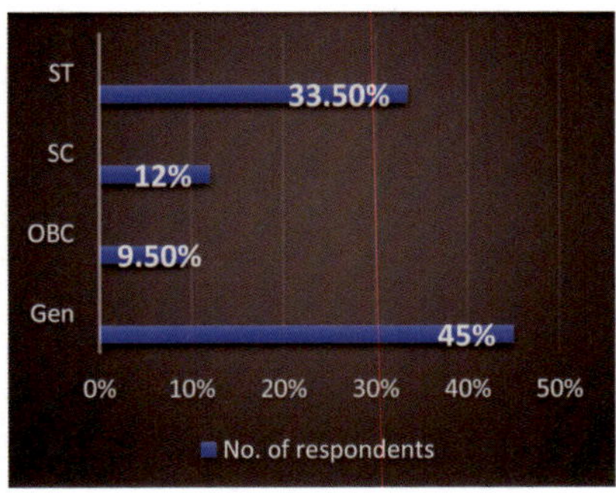


**Fig. 6.** Social Status

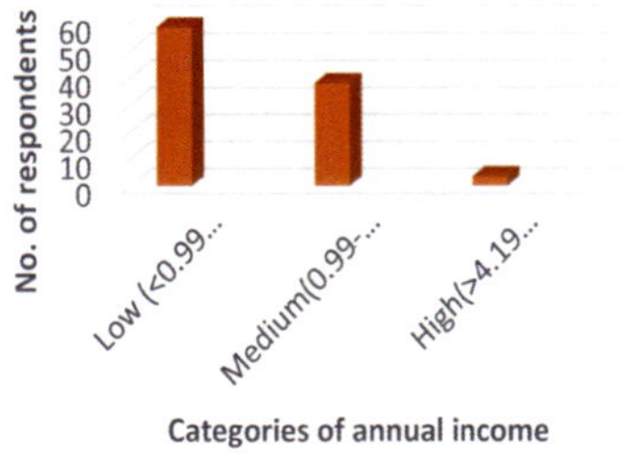


**Fig. 7.** Annual Income (in Rs)

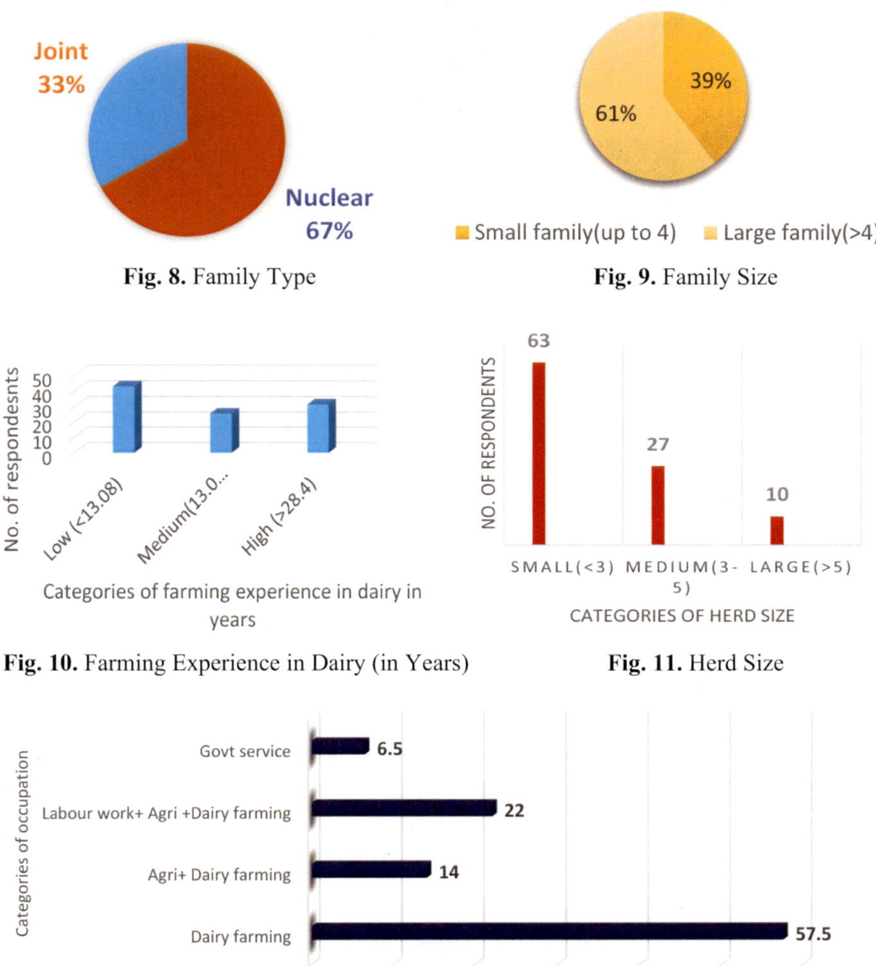


**Fig. 8.** Family Type

**Fig. 9.** Family Size

**Fig. 10.** Farming Experience in Dairy (in Years)

**Fig. 11.** Herd Size

**Fig. 12.** Occupation

#### 4.2.1.1 Caste wise distribution of respondents according to differential role performed in breeding aspect of dairy farming

From the table 4.6.1, caste wise distribution of respondents according to differential role performed in breeding aspect of dairy farming has been shown. Under breeding aspect, in the first parameter 'choosing different breeds of animal'; 35.60 percent of the general caste respondents has actively participated in the task, whereas, only 26.90 percent of the respondents belong to ST farmer category regularly participated in the said activity. It is interesting to notice that 47.40 percent of OBC respondents and 62.50 percent of the SC respondents were regularly involved in the afore mentioned activity. It suggested that respondents who belonged to SC and OBC category were more involved in the activity than other communities of farm women due to their major inclination towards the dairy farming activity. In case of second parameter, i.e., 'contacting veterinary officials for A.I', it has been seen that 42.10 percent of the OBC respondents and 58.30 percent of SC category respondents regularly participated in the activity whereas, only 13.45 percent of the respondents from ST community participated regularly in the said activity. So, in this case also the participation of the OBC and SC respondents in the activity was much higher than other communities. In case of another parameter that is 'taking animal for natural service', it has been seen that 35.80 percent of ST community member were regularly involved in the activity than other community members. It suggested that, ST community respondents were less oriented towards A.I activity. In the case of consulting veterinarian for infertility management majority (54.20%) of the respondents belonging to SC community were more involved compared to other categories.

Hence, it can be concluded that respondents under SC category were actively involved in the breeding aspect as compared to other categories. The reason can be attributed to their higher level of engagement in dairy farming.

### 4.2.1.2 Caste wise distribution of respondents according to differential role performed in feeding aspect of dairy farming

From table 4.6.2, caste wise distribution of respondents according to differential role performed in feeding aspect of dairy farming has been shown. Under the feeding aspect, in the parameter "collection of feed and fodder", 44 respondents who fell under the general category, 40 respondents who fell under ST, 15 respondents who fell under SC and 10 respondents who fell under OBC respectively, were regularly carrying out the activity. In the case of "feeding the animal", 78 respondents falling under general category, 55 respondents falling under ST, were either often or regularly involved in the activity. On the other hand, it can be observed that, 22 respondents who fell under SC category and 13 respondents who fell under the OBC respectively, were either often or regularly involved in the said activity. In the case of "storage of feed and fodder" higher regular involvement was observed in SC community, where 62.50 percent respondents were regularly involved, while 57.90 percent of respondents falling under OBC category, 53.70 percent respondents falling under ST category and 50.00 percent respondents falling under general category respectively, were also regularly involved in the activity. Regarding "watering and feed supplement" majority of the respondents under each category were regularly involved in the activity

It can be concluded that majority of respondents under all the caste category were performing feeding aspect activities. The reason behind this can be due to the fact that majority of respondents were practicing dairy farming as their main occupation.

#### 4.2.1.3 Caste wise distribution of respondents according to differential role performed in marketing aspect of dairy farming

From the table 4.6.3, caste wise distribution of respondents according to differential role performed in marketing aspect of dairy farming, it can be seen that under the marketing aspect, in the parameter "selling of milk and milk products to the household" revealed that 25.00 percent respondents who fell under SC category carried the said activity regularly, while 21.10 percent respondents who fell under OBC category, 14.90 percent of respondents who fell under ST category and 7.80 percent respondents who fell under general category were also carrying out the activity regularly. The table also showed that percent of the respondent who never practiced the activity were seen to be higher, which indicates that respondents under all the four categories were not much involved in the selling of milk and milk products to the household level. In the case of "selling of milk to cooperatives", it can be seen that respondents under all the four categories were not much involved in selling of milk to cooperatives as the percentage of involvement were seen to be low, where only 16.60 percent respondents under SC category were regularly involved followed by 13.30 percent respondents under general category, 10.50 percent respondents under OBC category and 7.50 percent respondents under ST category respectively, were regularly involved in the said activity. Regarding the "selling of value added products", the table exhibited that majority (50.00%) of SC category were sometimes engaged in selling of value added products while the rest of the categories were having low involvement.

Hence, it can be concluded that majority of the respondent under General, ST, SC and OBC category were not much engaged in marketing aspect. The reason behind this could be attributed to their various household activities; usually selling of milk to the other household and cooperatives were done early in the morning and women were mostly engaged in their household chores leaving them no time for carrying out marketing aspect and the male members of the family carried out these activities. Regarding the value-addition of the milk products, majority respondents under the four categories were not involved in this activity because most of the respondents belonged to low milk production category and had small herd size, which results in less possibility for value addition of milk products.

### 4.2.1.4 Caste wise distribution of respondents according to differential role performed in health care aspect of dairy farming

From the table 4.6.4, caste wise distribution of respondents according to differential role performed in health care aspect of dairy farming, it can be seen that under the health care aspect, in case of parameter "care of diseased animal" and "care of pregnant cows" the table clearly depicted that majority (50.00%) respondents who fell under the SC category were regularly engaged in the said activity, while 42.10 percent respondents who fell under the OBC category were also regularly engaged in the said activities. It can also be seen that low percent of respondents under ST category were regularly involved in the given activity. In the case of "care of new born" 18 respondents falling under SC category were either often or regularly involved in the said activity, while 11 respondents falling under OBC and 37.80 percent of respondents under general category were either often or regularly engaged in the said activity. On the other hand, less regular participation had been observed in ST and general category as compared to OBC and SC category. In the case of "vaccination management" regular involvement was found to be low for all the categories, whereas majority of the OBC category respondents were sometimes involved in vaccination management. Under "deworming management", 41.70 percent and 35.60 percent of the respondents under SC and general category, respectively, were regularly carrying out deworming management, while the other categories involvement was found to be low.

Therefore, it can be concluded that, respondents under SC, OBC and general category were mostly involved in health care aspect of dairy animal, while the ST category were seen to be less involved. The reason behind this may be linked towards culture and religious belief of SC, OBC and general category farmers where they believe cow as their goddess, and regarding the "vaccination and deworming management", as the general category respondents were having good social participation which helped them to collect various information regarding this matter and as a result of that, their regular participation was seen to be higher than other communities.

**Table 4.6.1.** Caste wise distribution of respondents according to differential role performed in breeding aspect of dairy farming (N=200)

| Sl. No. | Activities | General(n=90) | | | | OBC(n=19) | | | | SC(n=24) | | | | ST(n=67) | | | |
|---|---|---|---|---|---|---|---|---|---|---|---|---|---|---|---|---|---|
| | **Breeding aspect** | 1 | 2 | 3 | 4 | 1 | 2 | 3 | 4 | 1 | 2 | 3 | 4 | 1 | 2 | 3 | 4 |
| 1. | Choosing different breeds of animals | 25 (27.70) | 24 (26.70) | 9 (10.00) | 32 (35.60) | 1 (5.30) | 4 (21.00) | 5 (26.30) | 9 (47.40) | 2 (8.35) | 5 (20.80) | 2 (8.35) | 15 (62.50) | 16 (23.90) | 22 (32.80) | 11 (16.40) | 18 (26.90) |
| 2. | Contacting veterinary officials for A. I | 24 (26.70) | 34 (37.80) | 7 (7.70) | 25 (27.80) | 3 (15.80) | 7 (36.80) | 1 (5.30) | 8 (42.10) | 3 (12.50) | 4 (16.70) | 3 (12.50) | 14 (58.30) | 27 (40.30) | 22 (32.80) | 9 (13.45) | 9 (13.45) |
| 3. | Taking animal for natural service | 42 (46.70) | 18 (20.00) | 8 (8.90) | 22 (24.40) | 5 (26.30) | 7 (36.80) | 3 (15.80) | 4 (21.10) | 4 (16.65) | 13 (54.20) | 3 (12.50) | 4 (16.65) | 26 (38.80) | 9 (13.50) | 8 (11.90) | 24 (35.80) |
| 4. | Consulting veterinarian for infertility management | 22 (24.40) | 35 (38.90) | 8 (8.90) | 25 (27.80) | 2 (10.50) | 4 (21.10) | 7 (36.80) | 6 (31.60) | 3 (12.50) | 4 (16.65) | 4 (16.65) | 13 (54.20) | 21 (31.30) | 20 (29.90) | 14 (20.90) | 12 (17.90) |

(1=never, 2=sometimes, 3=often, 4=regularly)
(Figures in the parenthesis indicate percentage)

**Table 4.6.2.** Caste wise distribution of respondents according to differential role performed in feeding aspect of dairy farming(N=200)

| **Sl. No.** | **Activities** | **General(n=90)** | | | | **OBC(n=19)** | | | | **SC(n=24)** | | | | **ST(n=67)** | | | |
|---|---|---|---|---|---|---|---|---|---|---|---|---|---|---|---|---|---|
| | **Feeding aspect** | 1 | 2 | 3 | 4 | 1 | 2 | 3 | 4 | 1 | 2 | 3 | 4 | 1 | 2 | 3 | 4 |
| 1. | Collection of feed and fodder | 2 (2.20) | 12 (13.30) | 32 (35.60) | 44 (48.90) | 0 (0.00) | 5 (26.30) | 4 (21.10) | 10 (52.60) | 0 (0.00) | 1 (4.20) | 8 (33.30) | 15 (62.50) | 6 (9.00) | 11 (16.40) | 10 (14.90) | 40 (59.70) |
| 2. | Feeding the animal | 0 (0.00) | 12 (13.30) | 25 (27.80) | 53 (58.90) | 0 (0.00) | 6 (31.60) | 3 (15.80) | 10 (52.60) | 0 (0.00) | 2 (8.30) | 7 (29.20) | 15 (62.50) | 0 (0.00) | 12 (17.90) | 17 (25.40) | 38 (56.70) |
| 3. | Storage of feed and fodder | 1 (1.10) | 11 (12.20) | 33 (36.70) | 45 (50.00) | 0 (0.00) | 5 (26.30) | 3 (15.80) | 11 (57.90) | 0 (0.00) | 1 (4.20) | 8 (33.30) | 15 (62.50) | 6 (9.00) | 9 (13.40) | 16 (23.90) | 36 (53.70) |
| 4. | Watering and feed supplement | 0 (0.00) | 14 (15.50) | 25 (27.80) | 51 (56.70) | 0 (0.00) | 6 (31.60) | 3 (15.80) | 10 (52.60) | 0 (0.00) | 2 (8.30) | 6 (25.00) | 16 (66.70) | 2 (3.00) | 10 (14.90) | 16 (23.90) | 39 (58.20) |

(1=never, 2=sometimes, 3=often, 4=regularly)

(Figures in the parenthesis indicate percentage)

**Table 4.6.3.** Caste wise distribution of respondents according to differential role performed in marketing aspect of dairy farming (N=200)

| Sl. No. | Activities | General (n=90) | | | | OBC(n=19) | | | | SC (n=24) | | | | ST(n=67) | | | |
|---|---|---|---|---|---|---|---|---|---|---|---|---|---|---|---|---|---|
| | Marketing aspect | 1 | 2 | 3 | 4 | 1 | 2 | 3 | 4 | 1 | 2 | 3 | 4 | 1 | 2 | 3 | 4 |
| 1. | Selling of milk and milk products to the household | 46 (51.10) | 20 (22.20) | 17 (18.90) | 7 (7.80) | 0 (0.00) | 13 (68.40) | 2 (10.50) | 4 (21.10) | 6 (25.00) | 7 (29.20) | 5 (20.80) | 6 (25.00) | 24 (35.80) | 23 (34.40) | 10 (14.90) | 10 (14.90) |
| 2. | Selling of milk to cooperatives | 31 (34.50) | 29 (32.20) | 18 (20.00) | 12 (13.30) | 7 (36.80) | 9 (47.40) | 1 (5.30) | 2 (10.50) | 10 (41.70) | 7 (29.20) | 3 (12.50) | 4 (16.60) | 38 (56.70) | 21 (31.30) | 3 (4.50) | 5 (7.50) |
| 3. | Selling of value-added products | 16 (17.80) | 39 (43.30) | 21 (23.30) | 14 (15.60) | 9 (47.40) | 6 (31.60) | 0 (0.00) | 4 (21.00) | 2 (8.30) | 12 (50.00) | 4 (16.70) | 6 (25.00) | 22 (32.80) | 30 (44.80) | 8 (11.90) | 7 (10.50) |

**Table 4.6.4** Caste wise distribution of respondents according to differential role performed in health care aspect of dairy farming (N=200)

| Sl. No. | Activities | General (n=90) | | | | OBC(n=19) | | | | SC (n=24) | | | | ST (n=67) | | | |
|---|---|---|---|---|---|---|---|---|---|---|---|---|---|---|---|---|---|
| | Health aspect | 1 | 2 | 3 | 4 | 1 | 2 | 3 | 4 | 1 | 2 | 3 | 4 | 1 | 2 | 3 | 4 |
| 1. | Care of diseased animal | 15 (16.70) | 22 (24.40) | 18 (20.00) | 35 (38.90) | 1 (5.30) | 7 (36.80) | 3 (15.80) | 8 (42.10) | 1 (4.20) | 5 (20.80) | 6 (25.00) | 12 (50.00) | 11 (16.40) | 26 (38.80) | 17 (25.40) | 13 (19.40) |
| 2. | Care of pregnant cows | 14 (15.60) | 25 (27.80) | 18 (20.00) | 33 (36.60) | 0 (0.00) | 8 (42.10) | 3 (15.80) | 8 (42.10) | 1 (4.20) | 5 (20.80) | 6 (25.00) | 12 (50.00) | 13 (19.40) | 25 (37.30) | 16 (23.90) | 13 (19.40) |
| 3. | Care of new born calf | 14 (15.60) | 22 (24.40) | 20 (22.20) | 34 (37.80) | 0 (0.00) | 8 (42.10) | 3 (15.80) | 8 (42.10) | 1 (4.20) | 5 (20.80) | 6 (25.00) | 12 (50.00) | 11 (16.40) | 26 (38.80) | 18 (26.90) | 12 (17.90) |
| 4. | Vaccination management | 29 (32.20) | 24 (26.70) | 17 (18.90) | 20 (22.20) | 3 (15.80) | 11 (57.90) | 2 (10.50) | 3 (15.80) | 3 (12.50) | 10 (41.70) | 9 (37.50) | 2 (8.30) | 40 (59.70) | 16 (23.90) | 7 (10.40) | 4 (6.00) |
| 5. | Deworming management | 15 (16.60) | 26 (28.90) | 17 (18.90) | 32 (35.60) | 2 (10.50) | 12 (63.20) | 3 (15.80) | 2 (10.50) | 1 (4.10) | 6 (25.00) | 7 (29.20) | 10 (41.70) | 26 (38.80) | 23 (34.30) | 12 (17.90) | 6 (9.00) |

(1=never, 2=sometimes, 3=often, 4=regularly) (Figures in the parenthesis indicate percentage)

#### 4.2.1.5 Caste wise distribution of respondents according to differential role performed in housing aspect of dairy farming

From table 4.6.5, caste wise distribution of respondents according to differential role performed in housing aspect of dairy farming, it can be observed that under housing aspect, in the parameter "cleaning of cattle shed" the highest percent of respondents (83.30%) among SC category were regularly carrying out the said activity, followed by 63.30 percent respondents under general, 58.20 percent under ST and 52.60 percent respondents under OBC category, respectively. In the case of "construction of cattle shed" perusal of the table, revealed that respondents under all the four categories were not much involved in construction of cattle shed. In the case of "use of dung for manure" 70.80 percent and 63.20 percent respondents under SC and OBC category, respectively, were regularly using dung for manure. In the matter of "cleaning of animal before milking" the table showed that 83.30 percent of respondents under SC category were regularly involved in the said activity, while low participation of respondents were observed in ST category (28.40%). Regarding "milking of animal" 83.30 percent of respondents under the SC category were regularly engaged in the activity whereas, 34.40 percent of respondents under General category were engaged in the activity. It is interesting to notice that majority of the respondents under OBC category, were never carrying out milking of animal. In the case of "record keeping" the table showed that majority of respondents under all the four categories were not keeping the record of farm activities.

Therefore, it can be concluded that respondent under General, ST, SC and OBC categories were not actively involved in construction of cattle shed and were also not keeping the record of the milk. The reason behind finding is that, for construction they were heiring labour as they were not skilled enough in construction activities. For keeping of record of farm activities, they didn't find it necessity as well as understand the importance of record keeping. Majority of SC, OBC and General category respondent were actively involved in cleaning, milking and use of manure of the animals compared to the ST respondents because the activities might be considered as their daily household chores as most of the respondents were dairy farmers by profession.

**Table 4.6.5.** Caste wise distribution of respondents according to differential role performed in housing aspect of dairy farming (N=200)

| Sl. No. | Activities | General (n=90) | | | | OBC (n=19) | | | | SC (n=24) | | | | ST (n=67) | | | |
|---|---|---|---|---|---|---|---|---|---|---|---|---|---|---|---|---|---|
| | Housing aspect | 1 | 2 | 3 | 4 | 1 | 2 | 3 | 4 | 1 | 2 | 3 | 4 | 1 | 2 | 3 | 4 |
| 1. | Cleaning of the cattle shed | 2 (2.30) | 9 (10.00) | 22 (24.40) | 57 (63.30) | 1 (5.30) | 5 (26.30) | 3 (15.80) | 10 (52.60) | 0 (0.00) | 1 (4.20) | 3 (12.50) | 20 (83.30) | 5 (7.50) | 8 (11.90) | 15 (22.40) | 39 (58.20) |
| 2. | Construction of cattle shed | 53 (58.90) | 37 (41.10) | 0 (0.00) | 0 (0.00) | 13 (68.40) | 4 (21.10) | 0 (0.00) | 2 (10.50) | 10 (41.70) | 9 (37.50) | 5 (20.80) | 0 (0.00) | 43 (64.20) | 21 (31.30) | 1 (1.50) | 2 (3.00) |
| 3. | Use of dung for manure | 5 (5.60) | 14 (15.50) | 30 (33.30) | 41 (45.60) | 3 (15.80) | 0 (0.00) | 4 (21.00) | 12 (63.20) | 3 (12.50) | 2 (8.35) | 2 (8.35) | 17 (70.80) | 8 (11.90) | 12 (17.90) | 14 (20.90) | 33 (49.30) |
| 4. | Cleaning of animal before milking | 25 (27.80) | 21 (23.30) | 13 (14.50) | 31 (34.40) | 10 (52.60) | 1 (5.30) | 2 (10.50) | 6 (31.60) | 1 (4.20) | 0 (0.00) | 3 (12.50) | 20 (83.30) | 15 (22.40) | 22 (32.80) | 11 (16.40) | 19 (28.40) |
| 5. | Milking of animal | 25 (27.80) | 21 (23.30) | 13 (14.50) | 31 (34.40) | 10 (52.60) | 1 (5.30) | 2 (10.50) | 6 (31.60) | 1 (4.20) | 0 (0.00) | 3 (12.50) | 20 (83.30) | 15 (22.40) | 22 (32.80) | 14 (20.90) | 16 (23.90) |
| 6. | Record keeping | 54 (60.00) | 33 (36.70) | 2 (2.20) | 1 (1.10) | 14 (73.70) | 5 (26.30) | 0 (0.00) | 0 (0.00) | 8 (33.30) | 15 (62.50) | 0 (0.00) | 1 (4.20) | 38 (56.70) | 29 (43.30) | 0 (0.00) | 0 (0.00) |

(1=never, 2=sometimes, 3=often, 4=regularly) (Figures in the parenthesis indicate percentage)

**Table 4.6.6.** Caste wise distribution of respondents according to differential role performed in economic aspect of dairy farming (N=200)

| Sl.No | Activities | General (n=90) | | | | OBC (n=19) | | | | SC (n=24) | | | | ST (n=67) | | | |
|---|---|---|---|---|---|---|---|---|---|---|---|---|---|---|---|---|---|
| | Economic aspect | 1 | 2 | 3 | 4 | 1 | 2 | 3 | 4 | 1 | 2 | 3 | 4 | 1 | 2 | 3 | 4 |
| 1. | Taking loans for dairy animals | 24 (26.70) | 27 (30.00) | 13 (14.40) | 26 (28.90) | 9 (47.30) | 8 (42.10) | 1 (5.30) | 1 (5.30) | 6 (25.00) | 7 (29.20) | 9 (37.50) | 2 (8.30) | 36 (53.70) | 21 (31.30) | 6 (9.00) | 4 (6.00) |
| 2. | Insurance of the animal | 35 (38.90) | 45 (50.00) | 7 (7.80) | 3 (3.30) | 9 (47.30) | 8 (42.10) | 1 (5.30) | 1 (5.30) | 10 (41.70) | 14 (58.30) | 0 (0.00) | 0 (0.00) | 40 (59.70) | 24 (35.80) | 2 (3.00) | 1 (1.50) |
| 3. | Sale of the cattle | 23 (25.60) | 30 (33.30) | 20 (22.20) | 17 (18.90) | 6 (31.60) | 6 (31.50) | 1 (5.30) | 6 (31.60) | 10 (41.70) | 9 (37.50) | 1 (4.20) | 4 (16.60) | 27 (40.30) | 28 (41.70) | 6 (9.00) | 6 (9.00) |
| 4. | Purchase of cattle | 22 (24.40) | 33 (36.70) | 18 (20.00) | 17 (18.90) | 9 (47.30) | 3 (15.80) | 1 (5.30) | 6 (31.60) | 10 (41.70) | 9 (37.50) | 1 (4.20) | 4 (16.60) | 27 (40.30) | 28 (41.70) | 6 (9.00) | 6 (9.00) |

**Table 4.6.7.** Caste wise distribution of respondents according to differential role performed in decision making aspect of dairy farming (N=200)

| Sl. No | Activities | General (n=90) | | | | OBC(n=19) | | | | SC(n=24) | | | | | | | |
|---|---|---|---|---|---|---|---|---|---|---|---|---|---|---|---|---|---|
| | Decision making aspect | 1 | 2 | 3 | 4 | 1 | 2 | 3 | 4 | 1 | 2 | 3 | 4 | 1 | 2 | 3 | 4 |
| 1. | Expansion of the farm | 23 (25.60) | 29 (32.20) | 18 (20.00) | 20 (22.20) | 8 (42.10) | 4 (21.10) | 5 (26.30) | 2 (10.50) | 3 (12.50) | 9 (37.50) | 8 (33.30) | 4 (16.70) | 25 (37.30) | 33 (49.30) | 6 (8.90) | 3 (4.50) |
| 2. | Adopting new farm technologies | 34 (37.70) | 26 (28.90) | 15 (16.70) | 15 (16.70) | 5 (26.30) | 7 (36.90) | 5 (26.30) | 2 (10.50) | 6 (25.00) | 8 (33.40) | 5 (20.80) | 5 (20.80) | 28 (41.80) | 25 (37.30) | 12 (17.90) | 2 (3.00) |
| 3. | Preparation of milk products | 4 (4.50) | 35 (38.90) | 20 (22.20) | 31 (34.40) | 6 (31.60) | 8 (42.10) | 5 (26.30) | 0 (0.00) | 2 (8.30) | 9 (37.50) | 2 (8.30) | 11 (45.90) | 23 (34.30) | 21 (31.30) | 8 (12.00) | 15 (22.40) |

(1=never, 2=sometimes, 3=often, 4=regularly) (Figures in the parenthesis indicate percentage)

**4.2.1.6** Caste wise distribution of respondents according to differential role performed in economic aspect of dairy farming

From the table 4.6.6, caste wise distribution of respondents according to differential role performed in economic aspect of dairy farming, it can be viewed that under economic aspect, in the parameter "taking loans for dairy animals", very less participation was observed among SC, OBC and ST respondents while 28.90 percent respondents under general category were regularly taking loans for dairy animals. In the case of "insurance of animal" the table revealed that respondents under all the four categories were not taking insurance of the animal on regular basis. The reason for this might, be attributed to lack of knowledge and information regarding dairy insurance schemes by the respondents. Regarding "sale of the cattle and purchase of cattle" the table displayed that the mostly respondents belonging to General and OBC category were regularly involved in the given activity, while ST category respondents were having low participation.

Therefore, it can be concluded that respondent under General category was comparatively more involved in economic aspect as compared to other categories. The reason for this can be due to the fact that general category respondents had higher social participation leading them to various information about different paper works like, loans, etc and are more open towards seeking knowledge regarding various developmental activities as compared to the other categories.

**4.2.1.7** Caste wise distribution of respondents according to differential role performed in decision making aspect of dairy farming

From table 4.6.7, caste wise distribution of respondents according to differential role performed in decision making aspect of dairy farming, it can be observed that under decision making aspect, the parameter "expansion of the farm", the table revealed that overall respondents were not much involved in decision making aspect as only 22.20 percent respondents under general category were regularly involved in decision making of expansion of the farm, while the role of other categories was seen to be very low. In the case of "adopting new farm technologies", the table showed that overall, very less participation of the respondents in the said activity. Regarding "preparation of milk products" the table exposed that 45.90 percent and 34.40 percent respondents under SC and general category were regularly preparing milk products. It was interesting to notice that no respondents under OBC were regularly undertaking the activity.

Hence, it can be concluded that majority of the respondent were not actively involved in decision making aspect. The reason for this might be lack of knowledge and less inquisitiveness about new technologies among the respondents. Regarding the preparation of milk product, SC and general category people were slightly more involved because milk product was important dietary component in their traditional culture.

### 4.2.2 Distribution of respondents for differential role accomplished by women dairy farmer with respect to annual income

In present study efforts have been made to measure the differential role accomplished by women dairy farmers in breeding, feeding, marketing, healthcare, housing, economic and decision-making aspect with respect to their annual income.

#### 4.2.2.1 Annual income wise distribution of respondents according to differential role performed in the breeding aspect of dairy farming

From the table 4.7.1, annual income wise distribution of respondents according to differential role performed in breeding aspect of dairy farming, it can be seen that under breeding aspect, the parameter "choosing different breeds of animals", the table exposed that 42.80 percent of respondents under high income category were regularly carrying out the given activity, followed by 38.50 percent under low income category. In the case of "contacting veterinary officials for A. I", 29.10 percent respondents under low income category and 28.60 percent respondents under high income category were regularly involved. Regarding "taking animal for natural service", 30.30 percent of respondents under medium income category were regularly involved in taking animal for natural service, while it was interesting to notice that 47.00 percent respondents under low income category were never carrying out the said activity. In the matter of "consulting veterinarians for infertility management" the table exposed that 29.90 percent respondents belonging to low income categories were regularly consulting veterinarian for infertility management.

It can be concluded that respondent belonging to the all income category were almost equally, regularly involved in breeding aspect.

**Table 4.7.1** Annual income wise distribution of respondents according to differential role performed in breeding aspect of dairy farming (N=200)

| **Sl. No** | **Activities** | **Annual income (in Rs)** | | | | | | | | | | | |
|---|---|---|---|---|---|---|---|---|---|---|---|---|---|
| | | **Low (n=117)** | | | | **Medium (n=76)** | | | | **High (n=7)** | | | |
| | Breeding aspect | 1 | 2 | 3 | 4 | 1 | 2 | 3 | 4 | 1 | 2 | 3 | 4 |
| 1. | Choosing different breeds of animals | 24 (20.50) | 35 (29.90) | 13 (11.10) | 45 (38.50) | 20 (26.30) | 18 (23.70) | 12 (15.80) | 26 (34.20) | 0 (0.00) | 2 (28.60) | 2 (28.60) | 3 (42.80) |
| 2. | Contacting veterinary for A.I | 39 (33.30) | 34 (29.10) | 10 (8.50) | 34 (29.10) | 18 (23.70) | 30 (39.50) | 8 (10.50) | 20 (26.30) | 0 (0.00) | 3 (42.80) | 2 (28.60) | 2 (28.60) |
| 3. | Taking animal for natural service | 55 (47.00) | 28 (23.90) | 11 (9.40) | 23 (19.70) | 22 (28.90) | 22 (28.90) | 9 (11.90) | 23 (30.30) | 0 (0.00) | 3 (42.80) | 2 (28.60) | 2 (28.60) |
| 4. | Consulting veterinarian for infertility management | 31 (26.50) | 31 (26.50) | 20 (17.10) | 35 (29.90) | 17 (22.40) | 29 (38.10) | 11 (14.50) | 19 (25.00) | 0 (0.00) | 3 (42.80) | 2 (28.60) | 2 (28.60) |

**Table 4.7.2** Annual income wise distribution of respondents according to differential role performed in feeding aspect of dairy farming (N=200)

| **Sl. No** | **Activities** | **Annual Income (in Rs)** | | | | | | | | | | | |
|---|---|---|---|---|---|---|---|---|---|---|---|---|---|
| | | **Low (n=117)** | | | | **Medium (n=76)** | | | | **High (n=7)** | | | |
| | Feeding aspect | 1 | 2 | 3 | 4 | 1 | 2 | 3 | 4 | 1 | 2 | 3 | 4 |
| 1. | Collection of feed and fodder | 5 (4.30) | 18 (15.40) | 30 (25.60) | 64 (54.70) | 2 (2.70) | 9 (11.80) | 22 (28.90) | 43 (56.60) | 1 (14.20) | 2 (28.60) | 2 (28.60) | 2 (28.60) |
| 2. | Feeding the animal | 0 (0.00) | 20 (17.10) | 30 (25.60) | 67 (57.30) | 0 (0.00) | 10 (13.20) | 21 (27.60) | 45 (59.20) | 0 (0.00) | 2 (28.60) | 1 (14.30) | 4 (57.10) |
| 3. | Storage of feed and fodder | 4 (3.40) | 15 (12.80) | 34 (29.10) | 64 (54.70) | 2 (2.70) | 9 (11.80) | 25 (32.90) | 40 (52.60) | 1 (14.30) | 2 (28.60) | 1 (14.30) | 3 (42.80) |
| 4. | Watering and feed supplement | 2 (1.70) | 18 (15.40) | 30 (25.60) | 67 (57.30) | 0 (0.00) | 12 (15.80) | 19 (25.00) | 45 (59.20) | 0 (0.00) | 2 (28.60) | 1 (14.30) | 4 (57.10) |

(1=never, 2=sometimes, 3=often, 4=regularly)(Figures in the parenthesis indicate percentage)

#### 4.2.2.2 Annual income wise distribution of respondents according to differential role performed in the feeding aspect of dairy farming

From the table 4.7.2, annual income wise distribution of respondents according to differential role performed in feeding aspect of dairy farming, it can be observed that, under the feeding aspect, in the parameter "collection of feed and fodder" the table showed that, 56.60 percent respondents under medium income category were regularly carrying out collection of feed and fodder. In case of low income category, 54.70 percent respondents were regularly undertaking the activity of collection of feed and fodder, in case of high income category only 28.60 percent respondents were regularly carrying out the said activity. In the case of "feeding the animal" the table revealed that majority of the respondents under all income categories were regularly involved in feeding the animal. In the case of "storage of feed and fodder" the table exhibited that majority of respondents under the low and medium income group were regularly undertaking storage of feed and fodder activity, while under the high income category 42.80 percent respondents were regularly undertaking storage of feed and fodder. Regarding "watering and feed supplement" the table showed that majority of the respondents under all categories were regularly involved in the activity.

Thus, it can be said that mostly the respondent under all the income category were actively involved in performing the roles under feeding aspect, except under the collection of feed and fodder the respondent under high income category were seen to be low as they prefer hiring labor for performing the activity.

#### 4.2.2.3 Annual income wise distribution of respondents according to differential role performed in the marketing aspect of dairy farming

From the table 4.7.3, annual income wise distribution of respondents according to differential role performed in marketing aspect of dairy farming, it can be seen that under marketing aspect, in the parameter "selling of milk and milk products to the household" very less regular participation was observed among respondents belonging to all the three income categories. It can be seen that 41.90 percent and 34.20 percent of respondents under low and medium income categories, respectively, were never involved in the said activity. In the case of "selling of milk to cooperatives", 43.60 percent and 43.40 percent respondents under low and medium income categories were never involved in the given activity, which proves that farm women were not regularly engaged in the selling of milk to the cooperatives. In case of "selling of value added products", 47.00 percent respondents under low income category, 39.50 percent respondents under medium income and 28.60 percent respondents under high income category were sometimes involved in the said activity, while very low percent of respondents were regularly involved in the activity. Therefore, it can be concluded that, few numbers of respondents irrespective of their income were regularly engaged in marketing aspect. The reason for this might be attributed to the fact that selling of milk and milk product were carried out mostly by the male member in the family.

#### 4.2.2.4 Annual income wise distribution of respondents according to differential role performed in the health care aspect of dairy farming

From table 4.7.4, annual income wise distribution of respondents according to differential role performed in health care aspect of dairy farming, it was observed under health care aspect, in the parameter "care of diseased animal" and "care of pregnant cow", 42.10 percent respondents each belonging to medium income group were regularly engaged in the said activities, while majority of the respondents under high income category were never involved in the said activities. On the other hand, 29.10 percent and 23.40 percent respondents belonging to low income category were regularly taking care of diseased animal and care of pregnant cow. In the case of "care of new born", 42.10 percent respondents belonging to medium income category were regularly engaged in the activity, while majority of the respondents under high income group were never engaged in the given activity. In the matter of "vaccination management", 71.40 percent respondent under high income category were never involved in vaccination management followed by 42.70 percent respondents under low income category and 26.30 percent under medium income category, respectively, were never involved in the said activity. Regarding the parameter "deworming management", 31.60 percent respondents under medium income category were regularly engaged in the activity followed by 28.60 percent under high income group were regularly engaged, while very few respondents under low income group were regularly engaged in the activity. Thus, it can be concluded that under health care aspect all the income categories were actively involved except for vaccination and deworming management, the low income group showed low involvement. The reason for the low income respondent's low involvement in the activities may be attribute to lack of awareness related to health care aspect and limited training facility on disease management activities.

**Table 4.7.3** Annual income wise distribution of respondents according to differential role performed in marketing aspect of dairy farming (N=200)

| Sl. No | Activities | Annual Income (in Rs) | | | | | | | | | | | |
|---|---|---|---|---|---|---|---|---|---|---|---|---|---|
| | | Low (n=117) | | | | Medium (n=76) | | | | High (n=7) | | | |
| | Marketing aspect | 1 | 2 | 3 | 4 | 1 | 2 | 3 | 4 | 1 | 2 | 3 | 4 |
| 1. | Selling of milk and milk products to the household | 49 (41.90) | 36 (30.80) | 15 (12.80) | 17 (14.50) | 26 (34.20) | 26 (34.20) | 15 (19.70) | 9 (11.90) | 1 (14.30) | 1 (14.30) | 4 (57.10) | 1 (14.30) |
| 2. | Selling of milk to cooperatives | 51 (43.60) | 40 (34.10) | 12 (10.30) | 14 (12.00) | 33 (43.40) | 23 (30.30) | 12 (15.80) | 8 (10.50) | 2 (28.60) | 3 (42.80) | 1 (14.30) | 1 (14.30) |
| 3. | Selling of value-added products | 26 (22.20) | 55 (47.00) | 16 (13.70) | 20 (17.10) | 20 (26.30) | 30 (39.50) | 15 (19.70) | 11 (14.50) | 3 (42.80) | 2 (28.60) | 2 (28.60) | 0 (0.00) |

**Table 4.7.4** Annual income wise distribution of respondents according to differential role performed in health care aspect of dairy farming (N=200)

| Sl. No | Activities | Annual Income (in Rs) | | | | | | | | | | | |
|---|---|---|---|---|---|---|---|---|---|---|---|---|---|
| | | Low (n=117) | | | | Medium (n=76) | | | | High (n=7) | | | |
| | Health care aspect | 1 | 2 | 3 | 4 | 1 | 2 | 3 | 4 | 1 | 2 | 3 | 4 |
| 1. | Care of diseased animal | 16 (13.70) | 42 (35.90) | 25 (21.30) | 34 (29.10) | 8 (10.50) | 17 (22.40) | 19 (25.00) | 32 (42.10) | 4 (57.10) | 1 (14.30) | 0 (0.00) | 2 (28.60) |
| 2. | Care of pregnant cows | 16 (13.70) | 41 (35.00) | 28 (23.90) | 32 (27.40) | 8 (10.50) | 21 (27.70) | 15 (19.70) | 32 (42.10) | 4 (57.10) | 1 (14.30) | 0 (0.00) | 2 (28.60) |
| 3. | Care of new born calf | 16 (13.70) | 42 (35.90) | 27 (23.00) | 32 (27.40) | 6 (7.90) | 19 (25.00) | 19 (25.00) | 32 (42.10) | 4 (57.10) | 0 (0.00) | 1 (14.30) | 2 (28.60) |
| 4. | Vaccination management | 50 (42.70) | 35 (29.90) | 19 (16.30) | 13 (11.10) | 20 (26.30) | 26 (34.20) | 16 (21.10) | 14 (18.40) | 5 (71.40) | 0 (0.00) | 0 (0.00) | 2 (28.60) |
| 5. | Deworming management | 30 (25.60) | 40 (34.20) | 23 (19.70) | 24 (20.50) | 10 (13.20) | 27 (35.50) | 15 (19.70) | 24 (31.60) | 4 (57.10) | 0 (0.00) | 1 (14.30) | 2 (28.60) |

(1=never, 2=sometimes, 3=often, 4=regularly)(Figures in the parenthesis indicate percentage)

### 4.2.2.5 Annual income wise distribution of respondents according to differential role performed in the housing aspect of dairy farming

From table 4.7.5, annual income wise distribution of respondents according to differential role performed in housing aspect of dairy farming, it can be seen that under housing aspect, the parameter "cleaning of the cattle shed", majority of the respondents under all the income categories were regularly undertaking cleaning of the cattle shed. Regarding the parameter "construction of cattle shed" the role performed by the respondents were found to be negligible. The reason can be due to lack of skill, experience in construction work. In the case of "using dung for manure" the table disclosed that majority of the respondents under low (51.30%), medium (50.00%) and high (71.40%) income category, respectively, were regularly practicing use of the dung for manure. In the matter of "cleaning of animal before milking" the table indicated that, 43.40 percent respondents belonging to medium income category and 35.90 percent of respondents belonging to low income category were regularly carrying out the activity while majority of the respondents under high income category were not involved in the activity as they used to hire labour for such activities. In case of "milking of animal", table displayed that 42.10 percent respondents belonging to medium income category and 34.20 percent respondents belonging to low income category were regularly milking animal. Low participation was observed under high income group. In the case of "record keeping" the respondent's participation was found to be insignificant; the reason might be due to lack of knowledge and negligence regarding the practice.

Thus, it can be concluded that medium and low income categories were mostly performing roles like cleaning of animal before milking and milking of animal etc. as compared to the high-income category. High income category respondents were engaging hired manpower for accomplishing those activities.

### 4.2.2.6 Annual income wise distribution of respondents according to differential role performed in the economic aspect of dairy farming

From the table 4.7.6, annual income wise distribution of respondents according to differential role performed in economic aspect of dairy farming, it can be observed that under economic aspect, the parameter "taking loans for dairy animals", majority (57.10%) respondents belonging to high income category were regularly taking loans for dairy animals while, only 15.40 percent of respondents under low income category were regularly involved in the given activity. In case of "insurance of animal", it can be seen that maximum number of respondents under all the three categories were never taking

**Table 4.7.5** Annual income wise distribution of respondents according to differential role performed in housing aspect of dairy farming (N=200)

| Sl. No | Activities | Annual Income (in Rs) | | | | | | | | | | | |
|---|---|---|---|---|---|---|---|---|---|---|---|---|---|
| | | **Low(n=117)** | | | | **Medium(n=76)** | | | | **High(n=7)** | | | |
| | Housing aspect | 1 | 2 | 3 | 4 | 1 | 2 | 3 | 4 | 1 | 2 | 3 | 4 |
| 1. | Cleaning of the cattle shed | 5 (4.30) | 12 (10.30) | 34 (29.00) | 66 (56.40) | 3 (3.90) | 10 (13.20) | 8 (10.50) | 55 (72.40) | 0 (0.00) | 1 (14.30) | 1 (14.30) | 5 (71.40) |
| 2. | Construction of cattle shed | 74 (63.20) | 36 (30.80) | 3 (2.60) | 4 (3.40) | 42 (55.30) | 31 (40.80) | 3 (3.90) | 0 (0.00) | 3 (42.90) | 4 (57.10) | 0 (0.00) | 0 (0.00) |
| 3. | Use of dung for manure | 13 (11.10) | 18 (15.40) | 26 (22.20) | 60 (51.30) | 6 (7.90) | 9 (11.80) | 23 (30.30) | 38 (50.00) | 0 (0.00) | 1 (14.30) | 1 (14.30) | 5 (71.40) |
| 4. | Cleaning of animal before milking | 31 (26.50) | 24 (20.50) | 20 (17.10) | 42 (35.90) | 16 (21.10) | 19 (25.00) | 8 (10.50) | 33 (43.40) | 4 (57.10) | 1 (14.30) | 1 (14.30) | 1 (14.30) |
| 5. | Milking of animal | 31 (26.50) | 24 (20.50) | 22 (18.80) | 40 (34.20) | 16 (21.10) | 19 (25.00) | 9 (11.80) | 32 (42.10) | 4 (57.10) | 1 (14.30) | 1 (14.30) | 1 (14.30) |
| 6. | Record keeping | 67 (57.30) | 49 (41.90) | 1 (0.80) | 0 (0.00) | 43 (56.60) | 32 (42.10) | 0 (0.00) | 1 (1.30) | 4 (57.10) | 1 (14.30) | 1 (14.30) | 1 (14.30) |

(1=never, 2=sometimes, 3=often, 4=regularly)

(Figures in the parenthesis indicate percentage)

**Table 4.7.6** Annual income wise distribution of respondents according to differential role performed in economic aspect of dairy farming (N=200)

| Sl. No | Activities | Annual Income (in Rs) | | | | | | | | | | | |
|---|---|---|---|---|---|---|---|---|---|---|---|---|---|
| | | Low (n=117) | | | | Medium (n=76) | | | | High (n=7) | | | |
| | Economic aspect | 1 | 2 | 3 | 4 | 1 | 2 | 3 | 4 | 1 | 2 | 3 | 4 |
| 1. | Taking loans for dairy animals | 53 (45.30) | 38 (32.50) | 8 (6.80) | 18 (15.40) | 20 (26.30) | 25 (32.90) | 13 (17.10) | 18 (23.70) | 2 (28.60) | 0 (0.00) | 1 (14.30) | 4 (57.10) |
| 2. | Insurance of the animal | 55 (47.00) | 54 (46.20) | 6 (5.10) | 2 (1.70) | 35 (46.10) | 35 (46.10) | 4 (5.20) | 2 (2.60) | 4 (57.10) | 2 (28.60) | 0 (0.00) | 1 (14.30) |
| 3. | Sale of the cattle | 42 (35.90) | 43 (36.80) | 12 (10.20) | 20 (17.10) | 15 (19.70) | 29 (38.20) | 14 (18.40) | 18 (23.70) | 3 (42.80) | 1 (14.30) | 2 (28.60) | 1 (14.30) |
| 4. | Purchase of cattle | 41 (35.00) | 43 (36.80) | 13 (11.10) | 20 (17.10) | 18 (23.70) | 29 (38.20) | 11 (14.40) | 18 (23.70) | 3 (42.80) | 1 (14.30) | 2 (28.60) | 1 (14.30) |

**Table 4.7.7** Annual income wise distribution of respondents according to differential role performed in decision making aspect of dairy farming (N=200)

| Sl. No | Activities | Annual Income (in Rs) | | | | | | | | | | | |
|---|---|---|---|---|---|---|---|---|---|---|---|---|---|
| | | Low (n=117) | | | | Medium (n=76) | | | | High (n=7) | | | |
| | Decision making aspect | 1 | 2 | 3 | 4 | 1 | 2 | 3 | 4 | 1 | 2 | 3 | 4 |
| 1. | Expansion of the farm | 40 (34.20) | 46 (39.30) | 18 (15.40) | 13 (11.10) | 17 (22.40) | 27 (35.50) | 15 (19.70) | 17 (22.40) | 2 (28.60) | 2 (28.60) | 0 (0.00) | 3 (42.80) |
| 2. | Adopting new farm technologies | 45 (38.50) | 41 (35.00) | 19 (16.20) | 12 (10.30) | 26 (34.20) | 24 (31.60) | 15 (19.70) | 11 (14.50) | 2 (28.60) | 1 (14.30) | 3 (42.80) | 1 (14.30) |
| 3. | Preparation of milk products | 26 (22.30) | 41 (35.00) | 22 (18.80) | 28 (23.90) | 7 (9.20) | 29 (38.20) | 13 (17.10) | 27 (35.50) | 2 (28.60) | 3 (42.80) | 0 (0.00) | 2 (28.60) |

(1=never, 2=sometimes, 3=often, 4=regularly)(Figures in the parenthesis indicate percentage)

insurance of animal. In the case of "sale of cattle" and "purchase of cattle", it can also be observed that 23.70 percent respondents under medium income category, followed by 17.10 percent respondents under low income category were regularly carrying out the activities, while low participation has been observed in high income category. Thus, it can be concluded that, the respondents were not performing an active role in economic aspect. Respondents belonging to low and medium income were slightly more involved in economic aspect than high-income category except for taking loans as majority of the respondent under high income category were taking loans for dairy animals. The reason can be attributed to the fact that low and medium income respondents were less educated and found it difficult in taking loans, insurance as it involves paper work while the high income respondents were possessing assets required for taking loans.

#### 4.2.2.7 Annual income wise distribution of respondents according to differential role performed in the decision making aspect of dairy farming

From table 4.7.7, annual income wise distribution of respondents according to differential role performed in decision making aspect of dairy farming, it can be viewed that under decision making aspect, in the parameter "expansion of farm", 42.80 percent of respondents under high income category were regularly engaged in the said activity, while low participation has been observed among the low and medium income group respondents. In the case of "adopting new farm technologies" very less regular participation was observed among respondents belonging to the all income categories which proves that farm women were reluctant in adopting new farm technologies. In the case of "preparation of milk products", 28.60 percent respondents under high income respondents and 35.50 percent respondents under medium income categories were regularly involved in the given activity. Thus, it can be concluded that, mostly medium income category and high income category were slightly more involved in decision making aspect as compared to low income category, which shows that respondents who belong to high income group were having more freedom towards decision making than low income group respondents.

## 4.3 Measurement of the magnitude of socio-economic empowerment of women dairy farmer of the study area

Through the study efforts have been made to measure the magnitude of socio-economic empowerment of women farmers engaged in dairying. Various socio-economic variables have been taken under consideration to measure the empowerment.

**Table. 4.8.1.** Distribution of respondents according to empowerment scores

| Sl. No | Empowerment scores | Frequency | Percentage |
|---|---|---|---|
| 1. | Low (<59.74) | 57 | 28.50 |
| 2. | Medium (59.74-80.74) | 70 | 35.00 |
| 3. | High (>80.74) | 73 | 36.50 |

From table, 4.8.1, it can be observed that 36.50 percent of the respondents were possessing high empowerment scores, while 35.00 percent were possessing medium empowerment scores. On the other hand, only 28.50 percent of the respondents were possessing low empowerment score.

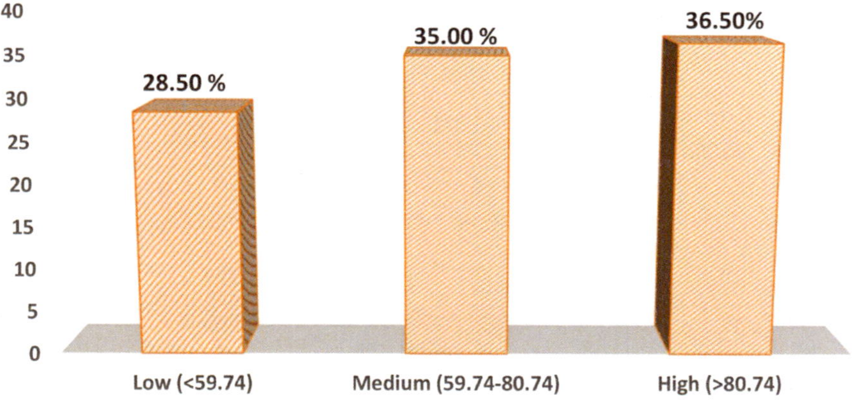


**Fig. 13.** Empowerment Scores of the Respondents

**Table 4.8.2.** Distribution of respondents according to empowerment scores with respect to different socio-economic variables (n=200)

| Sl. No | Variables | Categories | Empowerment Scores |
|---|---|---|---|
| | | | Mean ± SEM |
| 1. | Age | Young (up to 35) | $81.48^{a} \pm 1.46$ |
| | | Middle (36-50) | $79.70^{a} \pm 1.63$ |
| | | Old (>50) | $63.35^{b} \pm 1.71$ |
| 2. | Education | Illiterate (0) | $61.33^{a} \pm 1.80$ |
| | | Primary (1) | $74.57^{b} \pm 1.90$ |
| | | Secondary (2) | $80.64^{bc} \pm 1.96$ |
| | | Higher sec. (3) | $81.99^{cd} \pm 2.26$ |
| | | Graduate and above (4) | $87.56^{d} \pm 1.96$ |
| 3. | Marital status | Married (1) | $74.81^{a} \pm 1.20$ |
| | | Unmarried (2) | $75.30^{a} \pm 2.50$ |
| | | Widow (3) | $61.74^{b} \pm 0.92$ |

| 4. | Milk production/ day (in litres) | Low (<7 lit) | $74.62^{ab} \pm 1.41$ |
|---|---|---|---|
| | | Medium (7 -13.50 lit) | $76.55^{b} \pm 1.84$ |
| | | High (>13.50lit) | $67.83^{a} \pm 4.09$ |
| 5. | Social status | General | $75.20^{ab} \pm 1.62$ |
| | | OBC | $81.46^{b} \pm 3.68$ |
| | | SC | $68.75^{a} \pm 3.80$ |
| | | ST | $73.51^{a} \pm 1.10$ |
| 6. | Farming Experience in dairying (In years) | Low (<13.08) | $79.87^{a} \pm 1.41$ |
| | | Medium (13.08-28.40) | $74.25^{b} \pm 2.15$ |
| | | High (>28.40) | $67.25^{c} \pm 1.11$ |
| 7. | Herd Size | Small (<3) | $71.43 \pm 1.52$ |
| | | Medium (3-5) | $72.27 \pm 3.30$ |
| | | Large (>5) | $68.37 \pm 4.83$ |
| 8. | Annual income through dairying (in Rs) | Low (<0.99 lakhs) | $73.78^{a} \pm 1.47$ |
| | | Medium (0.99-4.19 lakhs) | $76.80^{a} \pm 1.60$ |
| | | High (>4.19 lakhs) | $60.39^{b} \pm 8.60$ |
| 9. | Occupation | Dairy farming | |
| | | Agri+ Dairy farming | |
| | | Labour work + Agri+ Dairy farming | |
| | | Govt service+ Dairy farming | |

Different superscript indicates significant difference at 5 percent level of significance

### 4.3.1 Distribution of respondents according to empowerment scores with respect to different socio-economic variables

#### 4.3.1.1 Age

From the table 4.8.2, it can be observed that young and middle age group were more empowered than the old age group as the empowerment scores were seen to be higher. The table also showed that the empowerment scores of young and middle age groups differed significantly from the old age group at 5 percent level of significance. Thus, it can be concluded that younger generations were more empowered than the older generation. This can be attributed to educational reform and technological advancement in the society. Similar results had been observed in findings of Batool and Jadoon (2018)

#### 4.3.1.2 Education

The table 4.8.2, revealed that empowerment scores were having direct relationship with higher education. It can be said that empowerment scores increased as the education qualification increased. The illiterate group were possessing lowest empowerment score whereas, the graduate and above group were possessing the highest scores. There was statistical difference between the illiterate and the primary educated group. Thus, it can be concluded that higher the education level more will be the empowerment scores. Similar results have been found in study of Redzuan *et al.* (2010), Das *et al.*, (2019) and Shanti and Murty (2019)

#### 4.3.1.3 Marital status

From the table 4.8.2, it is evident that married and unmarried category were possessing greater empowerment scores than widow category. The reason behind this can be due to the fact that widow women are often looked down by the society and considered weak. The table also showed that empowerment score of married and unmarried categories differed significantly from widow category. Similar results have been found in study of Redzuan *et al.* (2010).

#### 4.3.1.4 Milk production per day (in liters)

The table 4.8.2, exhibited that medium milk production category was possessing greater empowerment scores, followed by the low milk production category, while the high category had the least scores. Thus, it can be concluded that low and medium categories were more empowered, the reason behind this can be due to their active social participation in gram panchayat, SHG and cooperative society meetings. It can also be observed that medium milk production category differed significantly from high category. Low category was not showing much significant difference from medium and high category.

#### 4.3.1.5 Social status

From the table 4.8.2, the result conveyed that higher empowerment scores were found in OBC category followed by General and ST. Least scores were observed in SC category. It can also be viewed that, OBC category differed significantly from ST and SC category, while general category and OBC were not showing much statistical difference in empowerment level. From the table, it can be said that OBC respondents of the region possessed the highest empowerment, the reason can be credited to their developed social structure where empowerment of an individuals was encouraged in the community.

#### 4.3.1.6 Farming experience in dairying (in year)

The table 4.8.2, conveyed that low farming experience category were possessing high empowerment scores, followed by medium category, while low scores were observed in high category. The table also verified that each category differed statistically from one another.

#### 4.3.1.7 Herd size

From table 4.8.2, it is quite evident that medium herd size was having more empowerment scores followed by small and large herd size. The table also disclosed that there was no statistical difference between the three herd size categories at 5 per cent level of significance.

#### 4.3.1.8 Annual income through dairying (in Rs)

The table 4.8.2, revealed that medium income category was possessing more empowerment scores followed by the low income category. Least empowerment scores were observed in the case of high income category. The table also exposed that there was statistical difference between the low and medium annual income categories and high income categories. Similar results have been seen in the findings of Shanti and Murty (2019)

#### 4.3.1.9 Occupation

It can be observed from table 4.8.2, that respondents under government service + dairy farming were possessing more empowerment scores then other occupational categories. It can also be seen that respondent under the government service + dairy farming category differed statistically from other three categories.

### 4.3.2. Distribution of respondents according to socio-economic variables vis-à-vis empowerment scores

#### 4.3.2.1 Age

It is evident from the table 4.8.3, that 21.00 percent of total respondents who fell under middle age group and 13.00 percent of total respondents who fell under young age group were possessing high empowerment scores as compared 2.50 percent of total respondents who fell under old age group. Thus, it can be concluded that the middle and young age group were more empowered than old age group. The reason behind this can be attributed to the fact that the younger and middle-aged generation farm women were educated, open to new ideas and can make decision of their own choices. On the other hand, the old aged generation were deprived of education due to the societal norms which made them less empowered. The table also showed the chi square value of 73.84 which proved that there was a statistical relationship between the age and empowerment scores at 1 per cent level of significance. Similar result had been found in the research of Khan and Maan (2008), Sheikh *et al.* (2016)

**Table 4.8.3.** Distribution of respondents according to socio-economic variables vis-à-vis empowerment scores (n=200)

| Sl. No | Variables | Categories | Empowerment score | | | Total | Chi square value |
|---|---|---|---|---|---|---|---|
| | | | Low | Medium | High | | |
| 1. | Age | Young (up to 35) | 3 (1.50) | 25 (12.50) | 26 (13.00) | 54 (27.00) | 73.84** |
| | | Middle (36-50) | 10 (5.00) | 24 (12.00) | 42 (21.00) | 76 (38.00) | |
| | | Old (>50) | 44 (22.00) | 21 (10.50) | 5 (2.50) | 70 (35.00) | |
| 2. | Education | Illiterate (0) | 37 (18.50) | 16 (8.00) | 2 (1.00) | 55 (27.50) | 73.63** |
| | | Primary (1) | 14 (7.00) | 23 (11.50) | 21 (10.50) | 58 (29.00) | |
| | | Secondary (2) | 6 (3.00) | 13 (6.50) | 23 (11.50) | 42 (21.00) | |
| | | Higher sec. (3) | 0 (0.00) | 10 (5.00) | 14 (7.00) | 24 (12.00) | |
| | | Graduate and above (4) | 0 (0.00) | 8 (4.00) | 13 (6.50) | 21 (10.50) | |
| 3. | Marital status | Married (1) | 49 (24.50) | 59 (29.50) | 71 (35.50) | 179 (89.50) | 25.55** |
| | | Unmarried (2) | 2 (1.00) | 11 (5.50) | 2 (1.00) | 15 (7.50) | |
| | | Widow (3) | 6 (3.00) | 0 (0.00) | 0 (0.00) | 6 (3.00) | |
| 4. | Family type | Nuclear (0) | 36 (18.00) | 51 (25.50) | 47 (23.50) | 134 (67.00) | 1.69 NS |
| | | Joint (1) | 21 (10.50) | 19 (9.50) | 26 (13.00) | 66 (33.00) | |
| 5. | Family Size | Small Family (up to 4) | 15 (7.50) | 36 (18.00) | 28 (14.00) | 79 (39.50) | 8.36* |
| | | Large Family(>4) | 42 (21.00) | 34(17.00) | 45 (22.50) | 121 (60.50) | |
| 6. | Milk production/day (in litres) | Low (<7 lit) | 38 (19.00) | 47(23.50) | 46 (23.00) | 131 (65.50) | 7.17 NS |

| | | | | | | | |
|---|---|---|---|---|---|---|---|
| | | Medium (7-13.50 lit) | 13 (6.50) | 13 (6.50) | 24 (12.00) | 50 (25.00) | |
| | | High (>13.50lit) | 6 (3.00) | 10 (5.00) | 3 (1.50) | 19 (9.50) | |
| 7. | Social status | General | 24 (12.00) | 32 (16.00) | 34 (17.00) | 90 (45.00) | 12.53 NS |
| | | OBC | 4 (2.00) | 5 (2.50) | 10 (5.00) | 19 (9.50) | |
| | | SC | 12 (6.00) | 3 (1.50) | 9 (4.50) | 24 (12.00) | |
| | | ST | 17 (8.50) | 30 (15.00) | 20 (10.00) | 67 (33.50) | |
| 8. | Farming Experience in dairy(In years) | Low (<13.08) | 11 (5.50) | 33 (16.50) | 42 (21.00) | 86 (43.00) | 30.21** |
| | | Medium (13.08-28.40) | 14 (7.00) | 16 (8.00) | 21 (10.50) | 51 (25.50) | |
| | | High (>28.40) | 32 (16.00) | 21 (10.50) | 10 (5.00) | 63 (31.50) | |
| 9. | Land holding | Marginal (<1ha) | 53 (26.50) | 66 (33.00) | 71 (35.50) | 190 (95.00) | 1.35NS |
| | | Small (1-2ha) | 4 (2.00) | 4 (2.00) | 2 (1.00) | 10 (5.00) | |
| 10. | Herd Size | Small (<3) | 34 (17.00) | 45 (22.50) | 47 (23.50) | 126 (63.00) | 0.41 NS |
| | | Medium (3-5) | 17 (8.50) | 18 (9.00) | 19 (9.50) | 54 (27.00) | |
| | | Large (>5) | 6 (3.00) | 7 (3.50) | 7 (3.50) | 20 (10.00) | |
| 11. | Annual income through dairying (in Rs) | Low (<0.99 lakhs) | 35 (17.50) | 44 (22.00) | 38 (19.00) | 117 (58.50) | 6.16 NS |
| | | Medium (0.99-4.19 lakhs) | 18 (9.00) | 24 (12.00) | 34 (17.00) | 76 (38.00) | |
| | | High (>4.19 lakhs) | 4 (2.00) | 2 (1.00) | 1 (0.50) | 7 (3.50) | |
| 12. | Occupation | Dairy farming | 41 (20.50) | 39 (19.50) | 35 (17.50) | 115 (57.50) | 18.15* |
| | | Agri+ Dairy farming | 10 (5.00) | 11 (5.50) | 7 (3.50) | 28 (14.00) | |

| | | | | | | | |
|---|---|---|---|---|---|---|---|
| | | Labour work + Agri+ Dairy farming | 6 (3.00) | 16 (8.00) | 22 (11.00) | 44 (22.00) | |
| | | Govt service+ Dairy farming | 0 (0.00) | 4 (2.00) | 9 (4.50) | 13 (6.50) | |

**Significant at 1 percent level of significance *Significant at 5 percent level of significance $^{NS}$ Non-significant

(Figures in the parenthesis indicate percentage of total respondents)

### 4.3.2.2 Education

It can be observed from the table 4.8.3, that 18.50 percent of total respondents who fell under illiterate category were having low empowerment scores, while respondents having primary and above education level were having high empowerment scores. The table also presented chi square value of 73.63 which proved that education and empowerment were having significant relationship at 1 per cent level of significance. Similar results had been found in the study by Bharathamma G. U. (2005), Kaushal and Singh (2010) and Sheikh *et al.* (2016).

### 4.3.2.3 Marital status

The table 4.8.3, exhibited that majority i.e., 71 married respondents were highly empowered than unmarried and widow. The reason behind this might be attributed to the fact that married women were supported and motivated by their partners. The result also displayed, chi square value of 25.55 which proved that marital status and empowerment were having significant relationship at 1 per cent level of significance. Similar result had been obtained from the study of Sheikh *et al.* (2016) who found that marital status was having a negative but significant relation with empowerment.

### 4.3.2.4 Family type

From the table 4.8.3, it can be observed that 25.50 percent and 23.50 percent of total respondents who fell under nuclear family type were having medium and high empowerment scores as compared to 9.50 percent and 13.00 percent of total respondents who fell under joint family. Thus, respondents belonging to the nuclear family were more empowered than the joint family. Family type and empowerment were not statistically related. Similar findings had been seen in study of Das *et al.* (2019) and Damodar *et al.* (2016).

### 4.3.2.5 Family size

The table 4.8.3, represented that, respondents falling under large family size were more empowered than small family size. It can be observed that 22.50 percent of total respondents who resided in large sized family possessed high empowerment scores as compared to 14.00 percent of total respondents who fell under small family size. The chi square value of 8.36 suggested that family size and empowerment were statistically related at 5 per cent level of significance.

### 4.3.2.6 Milk production per day (in litres)

It can be noticed from the table 4.8.3, that 23.50 percent and 23.00 percent of total respondents who fell under low milk production category were possessing medium and high empowerment scores, respectively. The reason behind this might be due to the fact that low milk production leads to low income and to increase the income the respondents belonging to the low milk production category were participating in various developmental activities and training, making them highly empowered compared to high and medium category.

### 4.3.2.7 Social status

From the table 4.8.3, it can be observed that highest number of respondents (17.00% of total respondents) falling under general category was having high empowerment scores. On the other hand, highest segment of ST respondents (15.00% of the total respondents) fell in medium empowerment category. It can be interesting to say that, a greater number of respondents (10 respondents) from OBC category fell in high empowerment category than that of low and medium empowerment category combined. This suggested, there was a trend of OBC category farmers falling in high empowerment group than other categories. The chi square value of 12.53 proved that social status and empowerment were not statistically related. Similar findings have been seen in study of Das *et al.* (2019)

### 4.3.2.8 Farming experience in dairying (in years)

The table 4.8.3, showed that 21.00 percent and 10.50 percent of total respondents who fell under low and medium farming experience category, respectively, were possessing high empowerment scores, whereas 16.00 percent of total respondents who fell under high experience category were possessing low empowerment scores. This shows that high farming experience and empowerment were having a negative relationship. Thus, respondents belonging to low farming experience category had high empowerment scores followed by medium farming experience category. The table also revealed the chi square value of 30.21, which showed that farming experience and empowerment were statistically related at 1 percent level of significance.

#### 4.3.2.9 Land holding

From the table 4.8.3, it can be observed that 66 and 71 respondents, falling under marginal land holding category were possessing medium and high empowerment scores, respectively, whereas only 4 and 2 respondents, falling under small land holding category were possessing medium and high empowerment score, respectively. Thus, marginal land holders were possessing high empowerment score compared to small holders.

#### 4.3.2.10 Herd size

From table 4.8.3, it can be observed that 45 and 47 respondents, belonging to small herd size category were having medium and high empowerment scores, respectively, followed by 18 and 19 respondents belonging to medium herd size category respectively. Under the large herd size category, 7 respondents each were possessing medium and high empowerment scores. Thus, it can be concluded that respondent under small and medium herd size were more empowered than large herd size, though the chi square value of 0.41 proved that herd size and empowerment were not statistically related.

#### 4.3.2.11 Annual income through dairying (in Rs)

The table 4.8.3, showed that a significant portion i.e., 19.00 percent of total respondents falling under low income category were possessing high empowerment scores while 17.00 percent of total respondents falling under the medium income categorywere having high empowerment scores. It can be interestingto say that 0.50 percent of total respondents falling under the high income group were having low empowerment scores. This proved that medium and low income group were more empowered than the high income group. The chi square value of 6.16 proved that income and empowerment were not related. Similar results had been observed in the study of Rahman and Naoroze (2007)

#### 4.3.2.12 Occupation

The table 4.8.3, exhibited that 4.50 percent of total respondents belonging to government service + dairy farming category were possessing high empowerment scores, followed by 11.00 percent of total respondents belonging to "labour work +agri +dairy farming" category were also having high empowerment scores. It can be seen that higher segment i.e, (20.50%) of total respondents belonging to dairy farming category were possessing low empowerment scores, while 5.00 percent of total respondents falling under "agri +dairy" farming category were possessing low empowerment scores. It was also observed that under "government service + dairy farming category" none of the respondents were possessing low empowerment scores, which showed that government employees were highly empowered. The chi square value of 18.15 proved that occupation and empowerment were statistically related at 5 percent level of significance. Similar results have been found in the study of Kaushal and Singh (2010) and Damodar *et al.* (2016), where family occupation had a significant relation with empowerment.

### 4.3.3. Distribution of respondents according to block wise variation in empowerment scores

**Table 4.8.4.** Distribution of respondents according to block wise variation in empowerment scores

| Block | Empowerment scores |
|---|---|
| | Mean ± SD |
| Nandok | 70.24 ± 2.48 |
| Ranka | 71.62 ± 2.48 |
| Rakdong Tintek | 70.47 ± 2.48 |
| Khamdong | 73.05 ± 3.18 |

The table 4.8.4, shows that there was no statistically significant difference in empowerment scores among the four blocks i.e., Nandok, Ranka, Rakdong Tintek and Khamdong. From the table it can also be seen that Khamdong block were having highest empowerment scores followed by Ranka block and Rakdong Tintek block, whereas, Nandok block was having the lowest empowerment scores.

## 4.4. Feedback given by the respondents related to dairy farming

**Table 4.9.1.** Feedback with respect to economical aspects given by the respondents related to dairy farming

| Sl. No | Feedbacks | Total score | Garrett mean score | Mean Rank |
|---|---|---|---|---|
| A. | **Economical aspects** | | | |
| 1. | High cost of crossbred animal | 9978 | 49.89 | IV |
| 2. | High cost of concentrate, feed and fodder | 13743 | 68.72 | I |
| 3. | Difficulty in getting loans from bank | 11087 | 55.44 | III |
| 4. | Lack of schemes for purchasing milch cattle | 9059 | 45.30 | V |
| 5. | High cost of medicine for cattle | 7453 | 37.27 | VI |
| 6. | Low productivity of local breed | 11569 | 57.85 | II |
| 7. | Lack of transport facility for milk and animal. | 7232 | 36.16 | VII |

The table 4.9.1 showed, the ranking of feedback given by the respondents regarding economical aspects. It can be seen that; "high cost of concentrates, feed and fodder" had been given first rank with mean score (68.72). The reason behind this might be due to the fact that, the area for fodder cultivation was very limited and there was lack of availability of good fodder variety to the cultivators. The feeds were usually bought from outside the state making it costly for the respondents to purchase. Similar results have been seen in study of Shankar *et al.* (2017) and Patel *et al.* (2016). Availability of concentrates, feed and fodder should be provided to the respondents at a subsidized rate by the government. Followed by second rank given to "low productivity of local breed" with mean score (57.85). The reason behind this can be due to the fact that local breeds of the area were producing milk on an average 5kg/day resulting in low productivity. Comparable results have been found in the study of Adhikari *et al.* (2020). Suitable training on feed management can be conducted in the area to improve the productivity of breeds in the area. Third rank was given to "difficulty in getting loans from bank" with mean score (55.44). Similar results have been reported by Patel *et al.* (2015). As majority of the respondents were marginal land holder and less educated to apply for loans in the bank.

**Table 4.9.2.** Feedback with respect to technical aspects given by the respondents related to dairy farming

| **B.** | **Technical aspects** | **Total score** | **Garrett mean score** | **Mean Rank** |
|---|---|---|---|---|
| 1. | Lack of bulk milk cooler in the milk centre | 8390 | 41.95 | V |
| 2. | Lack of machine milking system | 11007 | 55.04 | III |
| 3. | Lack of training on scientific cattle management. | 11719 | 58.60 | II |
| 4. | Lack of awareness on disease management | 10668 | 53.34 | IV |
| 5. | Delayed service of animal health officials | 12173 | 60.87 | I |
| 6. | Problem in heat detection | 6032 | 30.16 | VI |

From the table 4.9.2, representing the feedback with respect to technical aspects, it can be seen that, first rank had been given to "delayed service of animal health officials" with mean score (60.87). Second rank was given to "lack of training on scientific cattle management" with mean score (58.60) and third rank was given to "lack of machine milking system" with mean score (55.04). The reason behind this is due to, lack of availability of veterinary clinics at each village and lesser number of veterinarians. The state being an organic state, focuses more on agricultural activities, thus there is limited emphasis on scientific training on dairy management. Apart from that, the majority of the respondent possesses small herd size and belongs to low income category therefore, availability of machine milk in their household is not possible. Similar results have been found in the research of Singh *et al.*, (2019) and Shankar *et al.* (2017)

**Table 4.9.3.** Feedback with respect to administrative aspects given by the respondents related to dairy farming

| C. | Administrative aspects | Total score | Garrett mean score | Mean Rank |
|---|---|---|---|---|
| 1. | Lack of financial support from govt. | 13215 | 66.08 | I |
| 2. | Lack of veterinarian service in the village | 9400 | 47.00 | III |
| 3. | Lack of schemes promoting dairy farming | 10255 | 51.28 | II |
| 4. | Lack of training availability on new technology to the farmers | 8860 | 44.30 | IV |
| 5. | Lack of extension contacts in the village | 8275 | 41.38 | V |

From the table 4.9.3, showing the feedback with respect to administrative aspects, it can be observed that, the first rank had been assigned to "lack of financial support from government" with mean score (66.08). Followed by second rank assigned to "lack of schemes promoting dairy farming" with mean score (51.28) and third rank assigned to "lack of veterinarian service" in the village with mean score (47.00). Similar findings have been reported by Patel *et al.* (2015) and Hundal *et al.* (2015). The reason for this might be that, the administrative setup in the study area has no proper plan and programmes for implementing dairy related schemes and developmental activities.

**Table 4.9.4.** Feedback with respect to information networking aspects given by the respondents related to dairy farming

| D. | Information networking aspects | Total score | Garrett mean score | Mean Rank |
|---|---|---|---|---|
| 1. | Irregular information on govt. schemes on dairy | 13325 | 66.63 | I |
| 2. | Lack of information on new technology | 10035 | 50.18 | III |
| 3. | Lack of information on training of dairy practices | 11105 | 55.53 | II |
| 4. | Lack of information on disease and pest management | 9370 | 46.85 | IV |
| 5. | Irregular information on AI | 6165 | 30.83 | V |

From the table 4.9.4, showing feedback with respect to information networking aspects, it can be seen that, the first rank had been given to "irregular information on government schemes on dairy" having mean score (66.63). Second rank was assigned to "lack of information on training of dairy practices" having mean score (55.53). Similar findings have been reported by Patel *et al.* (2015) and Adhikari *et al.* (2020). The third rank was allotted to "lack of information on new technology" having mean score (50.18). The reason for this can be due to weak functioning of extension workers in the area, inappropriate communication technique and method followed by the officials and communication gap between the farmers and government officials.

**Table 4.9.5.** Feedback with respect to independence in decision making aspects given by the respondents related to dairy farming

| E. | Independence in decision making aspects | Total score | Garrett mean score | Mean Rank |
|---|---|---|---|---|
| 1. | Non availability of financial support to women dairy farmer | 12572 | 62.86 | I |
| 2. | Lack of knowledge on dairy activities | 7657 | 38.29 | IV |
| 3. | Poor managerial skills | 9808 | 49.04 | III |
| 4. | Lack of self-confidence | 9963 | 49.82 | II |

From the table 4.9.5, showing the feedback with respect to independence in decision making aspects, the first rank had been given to "non-availability of financial support to women dairy farmer" having mean score (62.86). Similar result has been in line with research of Hundal *et al.* (2015) and Fatima and Akhtar (2014) who found that financial empowerment was lacking in dairy women farmers. Second rank was given to "lack of self-confidence" with mean score (49.82). Similar result has been observed by Singh *et al.* (2017) and Dhayal and Mehta (2020) who reported that farm women were shy in nature and lacked self- confidenceand third rank was allotted to "poor managerial skills" with mean score (49.04). The reason behind this may be due to the fact that, majority of the respondents practiced agriculture and dairy farming as their occupation. They had no other source of income thus making them financially weak. Majority of the respondents possessed only primary education leading to lack of self -confidence and poor managerial skills.

# 5

# Glimpse of Data Collection

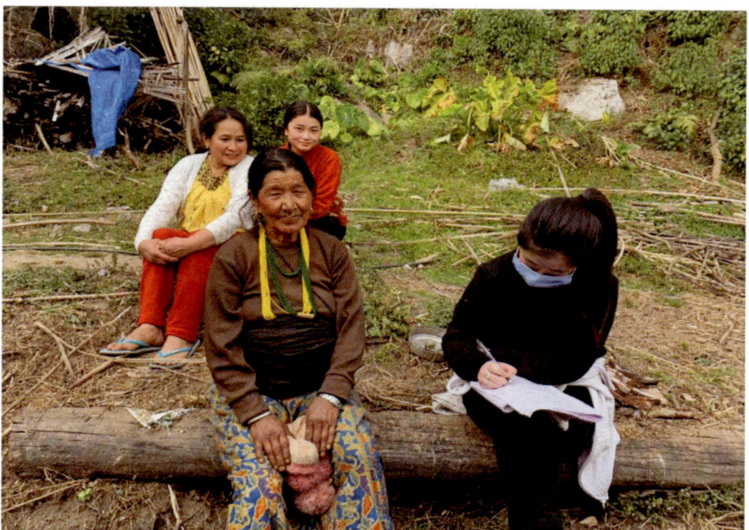

**Plate 1.** Personal interview with women dairy farmers

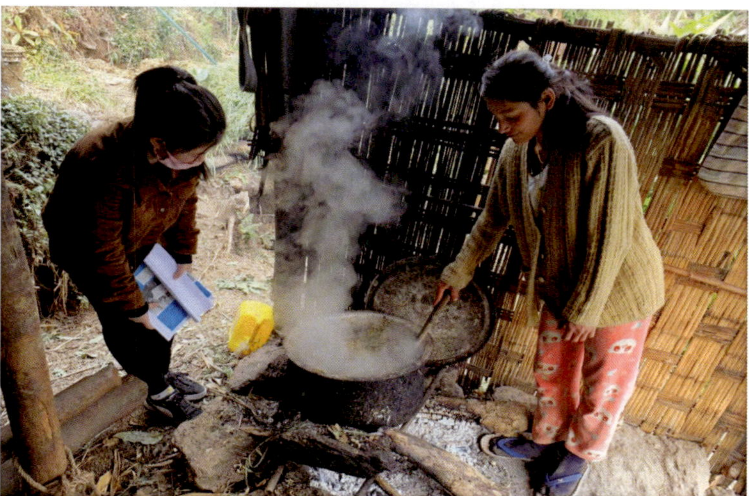

**Plate 2.** Preparation of feed by the respondent

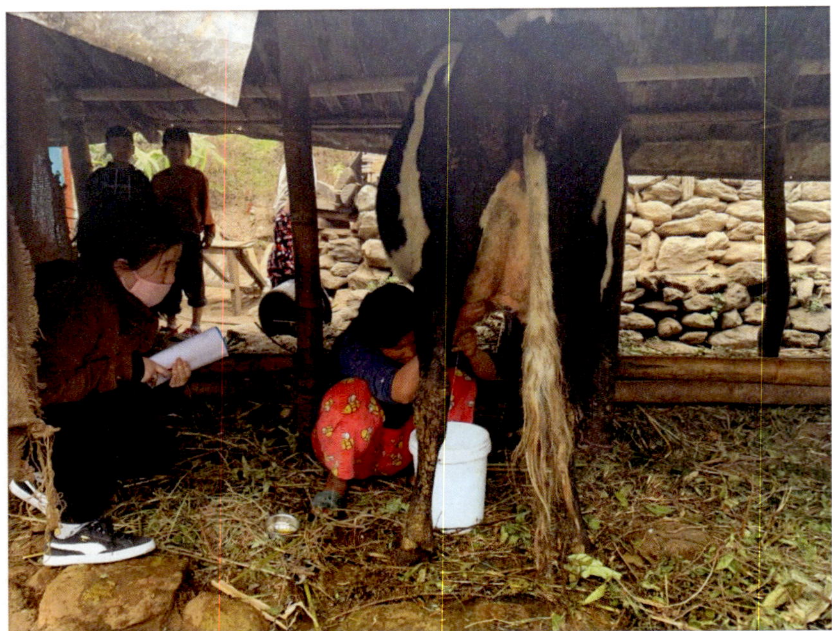

**Plate 3.** Milking of cow by the respondent

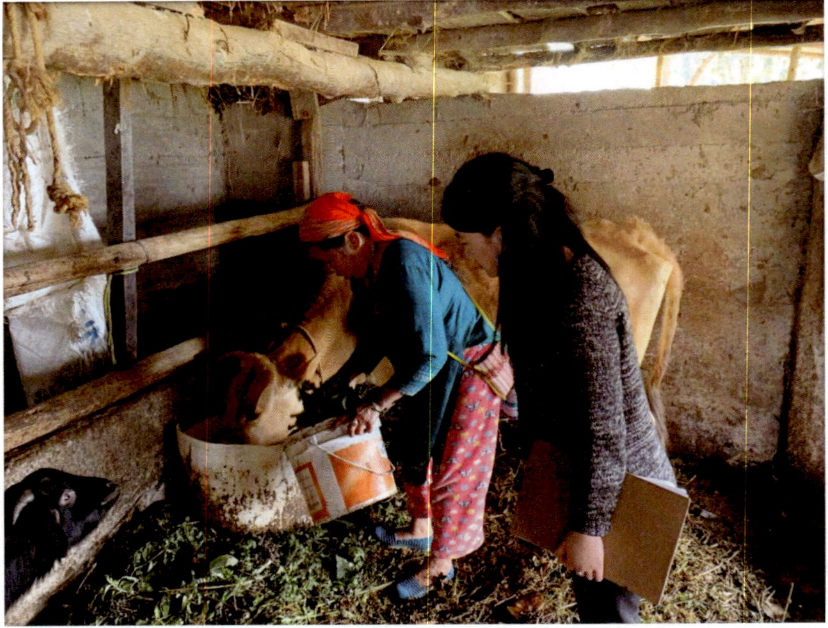

**Plate 4.** Respondent feeding of the animal

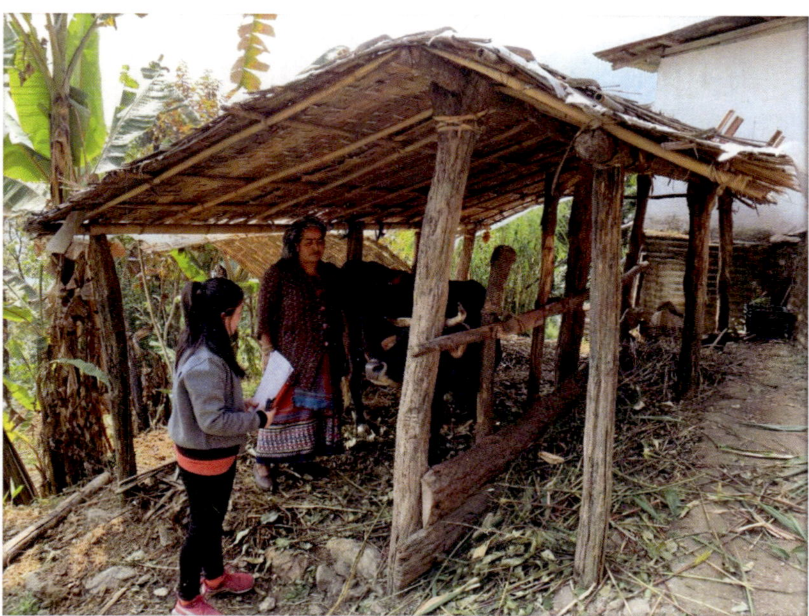

**Plate 5.** Traditional cattle housing system

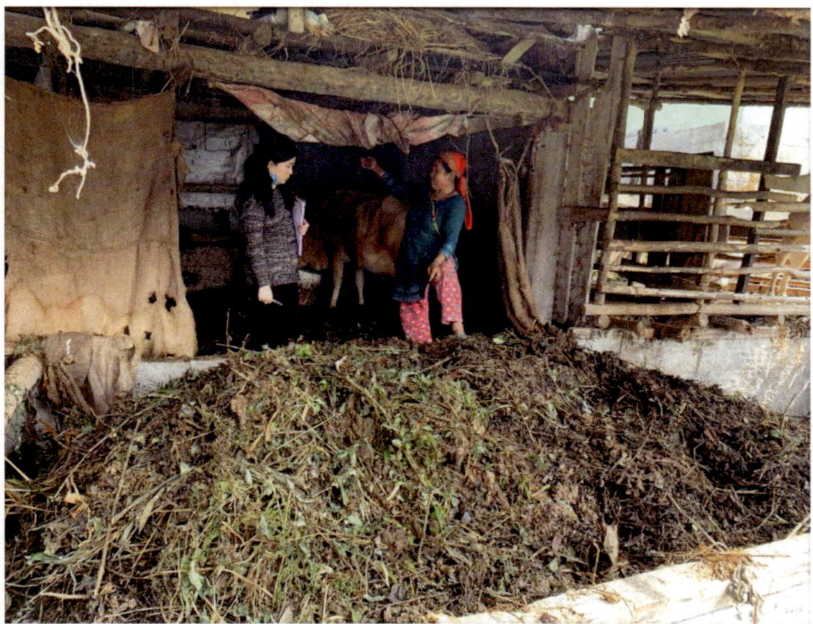

**Plate 6.** Use of dung for compost preparation by the respondent

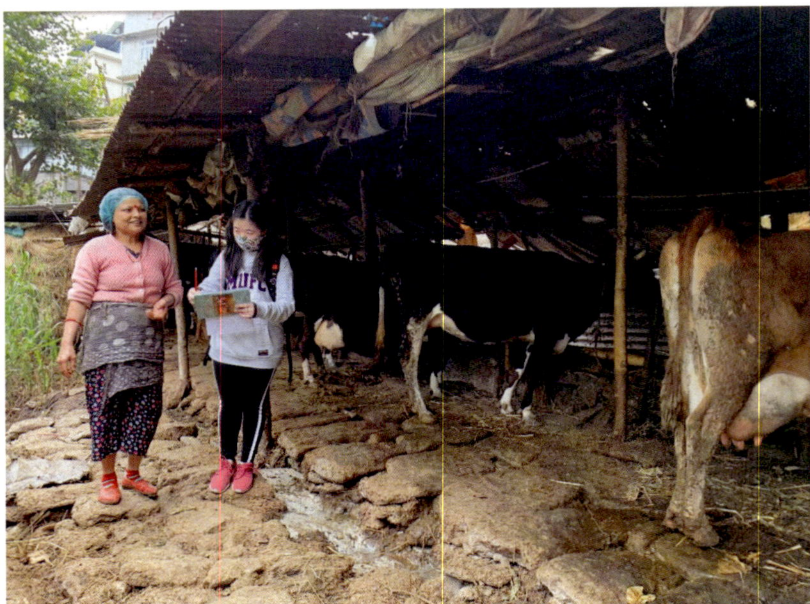

**Plate 7.** Recording feedback from the respondent

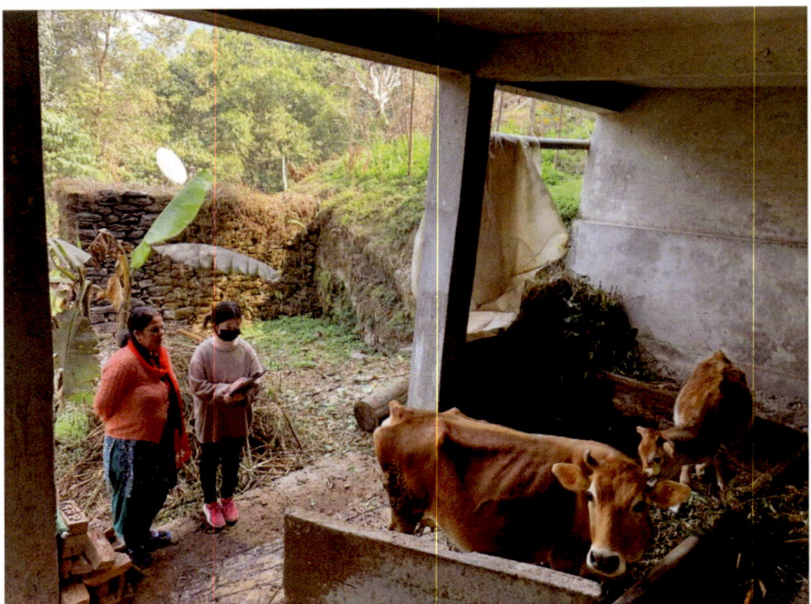

**Plate 8.** Farm condition for cattle rearing in the study area

# 6

# Summary and Conclusions

The contribution of dairy sector in the Indian economy has tremendous impact on the country's GDP. India being the world's highest milk producing country, dairy industry has a major role in changing the twin problem of the nation that is poverty and unemployment. Dairy sector also involves the under privileged group, especially the dairy farm women. There are many success stories regarding the life changing experiences gained by the farm women, who had taken dairy farming as a means to sustain their livelihood. In the area of gender equality, dairy sector has proved to be a women centric enterprise. Most of the activities pertaining to dairy farming are mostly carried out by the farm women. The dairy farming activities carried out by the farm women are tedious and in major cases their contribution remains unnoticed. They are usually carrying out activities, where most of their energy is drained, resulting in drudgery. Matters related to decision making, their opinion about adopting new technologies, starting an enterprise are not given importance by their family members. This leads to a greater setback in the emergence of success of dairy sector. Therefore, empowerment of farm women in dairy sector is one of the important criteria for the dairy industry to reach a greater height and for overall development of nation. With this background the study entitled **"Beyond the Milk Pail: Multidimensional Insights into Women's Participation in Dairy Farming in East Sikkim"** with the following specific objectives has been conducted:

### Objectives

1. To assess the differential role accomplished by women dairy farmers from different social strata in the study area
2. To measure the magnitude of socio-economic empowerment of women dairy farmer of the study area
3. To analyze the feedback of women engaged in dairying.

### 5.1 Research methodology

The study was undertaken in purposively selected East district of Sikkim. Four blocks were selected through random sampling technique. From each selected block, 5 villages were selected, and 10 dairy farm women were randomly selected from each randomly selected village. The total respondents for the study were 200. The data analysis was done by using statistical tools like frequency, percentage, chi-square test, ANOVA, ranking etc.

For the first objective of the study "To assess the differential role accomplished by women dairy farmers from different social strata in the study area", various dairy farming activities were taken into consideration. The activities were divided into breeding aspect, feeding aspect, marketing aspect, health care aspect, housing aspect, economic aspect and decision-making aspect. Under the various aspects, activities were presented as statements. The statements were categorized as regularly, often, sometimes and never, with scoring given as 4, 3, 2, 1. Cross tabulation was formulated for the various dairy related activities under each aspect with respect to caste and annual income from dairy farming of the women dairy farmers and frequency and percentage were taken into account.

For second objective "To measure the magnitude of socio-economic empowerment of women dairy farmer of the study area", an index was prepared by firstly selecting five dimensions namely, "Social Dimension", "Economic Dimension", "Freedom to mobility Dimension", "Technical knowledge possession Dimension" and "Decision making dimension". Under these dimension suitable statements were selected through secondary sources and were sent for judges rating in a google form format via emails. Expert in the field of women empowerment was selected as judges. The statements were also sent to the same judges to suggest the degree of relevancy of statements. Out of 150 judges, 58 responses were received and the means of the dimensions were calculated and weightage was taken. The relevancy weightage (RW) was calculated and the statement having more than 0.7 relevancy value were selected for index preparation. Total of 44 statements were taken in consideration under the five dimensions of empowerment. Weighted score for each dimension was calculated by multiplying the percentage scores of each dimension by their respective weights. It was done as (W1×SD), (W2×ED), (W3×FMD), (W4×TKD) and (W5×DMD). Socio-economic empowerment index (SEI), was obtained by adding the weighted score of each of the dimension of a respondent and then divided by 100. The categorization of the respondent on the basis of empowerment scores was done by using cumulative square root method. Chi square and ANOVA, Post hoc test was carried to measure the degree of association among various socio-economic variables with the empowerment scores.

For the third objective, "To analyze the feedback of women engaged in dairying". The feedbacks were presented to the respondent, which were classified according to economical aspect, technical aspect, administrative aspect, information networking aspect, independence in decision making aspect respectively. The respondents were asked to rank the statements given under each aspect according to the degree of importance as conceived by them.

## 5.2 Salient findings of the study

1. A total of 38.00 percent of the respondents belonged to middle age and 35.00 percent belonged to old age group.
2. It was found that 29.00 percent of the respondents were educated up to primary level and only 10.50 percent of the respondents were graduates.
3. It was found that 45.00 percent of the respondents were from general category, 33.50 percent were from Scheduled Tribe, 12.00 percent were from Scheduled Caste and 9.50 percent were from Other Backward Caste.
4. Most of the respondents (63.00%) possessed small herd size (less that 3 cattle), (58.50%) belonged to low annual income category with less than Rs 0.99 lakhs annual income and 48.00 percent respondents belonged to small livestock possession category.
5. Majority of the respondents (51.50%) were possessing building, 67.50 percent were taking money from informal source like, friends, neighbour and most of the respondents were participating in gram panchayat, cooperative society, SHG, religious gathering.
6. In case of time utilization pattern, 34.50 percent respondents were taking less than 1hour and 20 minutes in collection of fodder, 44.50 percent were taking 40 to70 minutes in feeding related activities, 42.50 percent were taking less than 30 minutes in cleaning of animal and cow shed, 40.00 percent were taking less than 15 minutes in milking cattle and 43.00 percent were taking less than 36 minutes in selling of milk.
7. From the differential role carried out by the respondents according to their caste in the study area, it was found that mostly SC category respondents carried out the activities related to breeding aspect, while majority of the respondents under all the categories were actively involved in feeding of the dairy cattle, and majority of the respondents under all the categories were not actively involved in marketing aspect of dairy farming.
8. 50.00 percent and 42.10 percent respondents belonging to SC category and OBC category respectively were regularly engaged in care of diseased and pregnant cows. 41.70 percent and 35.60 percent respondents

under SC and General category respectively, were regularly involved in deworming of livestock.

9. Majority of the respondents under all the four categories were involved in housing aspect particularly in cleaning of cattle shed, using of dung as manure.
10. General category respondents were mostly taking loans for the animals than other categories. Respondents under all the categories were not much involved in carrying out decision making aspect.
11. Majority of the respondents under all the income categories were carrying out activities under housing aspect, particularly cleaning of cattle shed and using of dung for manure.
12. 43.40 percent respondents from medium income and 35.90 percent respondents from low income category were mostly performing cleaning of animal before milking activity and 42.10 percent and 34.20 percent respondents under medium and low income categories were regularly engaged in milking of animal.
13. Majority (57.10%) respondents under high income groups were regularly taking loans for dairy animals.
14. 42.80 percent respondents under high income group were regularly taking decision regarding expansion of farm.
15. Socio- economic empowerment index in the study revealed that 36.50 percent respondents belonged to high empowerment category, 35.00 percent respondents belonged to medium category and 28.50 percent belonged to low empowerment category.
16. Young and middle aged, educated, married, medium income category respondents were highly empowered.
17. Age, education, marital status, farming experience in dairy, family size and occupation were having a statistically significant relationship with empowerment score. Family type, milk production per day, social status, land holding, herd size and annual income were not having any association with the empowerment scores.
18. Garret ranking technique was followed to measure the feedback given by dairy respondents and it was found that, high cost of concentrate, feed and fodder, delayed service of animal health officials, lack of financial support from government, irregular information on government schemes on dairy and non-availability of financial support to women farmers were some of the major feedbacks given by the respondents.

## 5.3 Conclusion of the study

The conclusion of the study are as follows:

1. Under the differential role accomplished by the women dairy farmers with respect to their caste, it was found that, SC category, OBC and General category respondents were involved in various aspect of dairy farming while the ST community were lacking behind, thus more proactive role of ST women farmers can uplift their social status.
2. General category respondents were mostly engaged in taking of loans for the dairy animal than compared to other communities. Ease of taking loans and availability of credit facility can help respondents from other communities to take loans for their purpose.
3. Respondents under all the caste category were actively involved in feeding aspect, while less involvement of all the respondents were seen in marketing aspect, thus marketing information may be provided to the respondents.
4. High income category respondents were mostly engaged in taking loans for the dairy animals than other categories, which suggested their economic orientation towards dairy farming. The respondents from other communities lacked in this aspect.
5. Respondents belonging to high and medium income groups were having more freedom towards decision making than low income group, which proved that with more income freedom in decision making maybe achieved.
6. The empowerment score of young and middle aged group were found to be higher than the old aged group. There was a significant difference in the empowerment scores among the young, middle aged group and old aged group.
7. Education was one of the important factors affecting empowerment as graduate and above respondents were more empowered that other categories of educational group in the study area.
8. Respondents from General and OBC categories, empowerment scores differed statistically with the empowerment scores of SC and ST category. OBC and General respondents were possessing high empowerment scores as compared to SC and ST category.
9. Major feedbacks given by the dairy women respondents were high cost of concentrate, feed and fodder, delayed service of animal health officials, lack of financial support from government, irregular information on

government schemes on dairy and non-availability of financial support to women farmers.

## 5.4 Implication of the study

The findings of the present study have presented some proposal in the manner of implication.

1. From the study the socio-economic empowerment of majority of the farm women was found to be in moderate to high level, the finding can be taken as an opportunity for implementing various dairy developmental program pertaining to upliftment of women in the state.
2. The result of measure of association revealed that age, education, marital status, family size, occupation and farming experience in dairy were some variables which were statistically related with the empowerment scores. Hence, the extension personnel should focus on these variables as they are enhancing the empowerment scores.
3. The extension personnel can conduct specialised trainings for the young women who were educated for taking dairy as their occupation. They can encourage married women to actively participated in SHGs, and provide trainings regarding value addition of milk and milk product to make them financially self-reliant.
4. Suitable schemes related to dairy development could be promoted among the ST communities for their upliftment in dairy sector in the study area, entrepreneurial development trainings can be provided to SC, General and OBC communities as these communities were showing active participation in dairy farming.
5. For strengthening the dairy cooperative and encouraging the entrepreneurial behaviour among farm women, the state should increase the price of raw milk.
6. The major feedbacks given by the farmers was high cost of concentrated, feed and fodder, the government should make an effort to formulated a scheme where the farmers may be provided with feed and fodder at subsidized rates. High yielding fodder varieties maybe popularised in the study area.

## 5.5 Suggestions for future research

1. The present study was conducted in East district of Sikkim. Only four blocks were taken in to consideration, resulting in limited sample size. Therefore, the generalization of the result cannot be made. In future, researchers can take a large sampling size for the study to be more universal.

2. Study should be carried out in depth on empowerment of dairy farm women in various region of the state.
3. The future researcher can include extra variables as per their interest to explore more about the topic.
4. In future, study can be undertaken to explore the entrepreneurial characteristics of dairy farm women of Sikkim.

# 7

# Bibliography

Adhikari, B., Chauhan, A., Bhardwaj, N. and Kameswari, V. L. V. (2020). Constraints faced by dairy farmers in hill region of Uttarakhand. *Indian Journal of Dairy Science*. **73**(5):464-470.

Agrawal, S. B., Singh, C. B. and Jha, S. K. (2007). Constraints in adoption of cross breeding technology in different regions of India. *Indian Journal of Dairy Science*. **60**(5): 360-363.

Anonymous. (2011). Office of RGI & Census commissioner of India, Ministry of Home affairs, Government of India.

Anonymous. (2011). Sikkim State Livestock Sector Policy: Perspective and Policy Elements. Government of Sikkim. Retrieved from http://www.sikkim-ahvs.gov.in/policy_final_4.pdf on 10-07-20

Anonymous. (2011). The role of women in agriculture. Food and Agriculture Organization. Retrieved from http://dahd.nic.in/about-us/divisions/cattle-and-dairy-development on 15-12-2020.

Anonymous. (2013). District-wise Breed- wise Cattle Population. Department of animal husbandry, dairying and fisheries, Ministry of agriculture and farmers welfare, Government of India. Retrieved from http://www.dahd.nic.in/animal-husbandry-statistics on 1-09-20.

Anonymous. (2016). Livestock Sector towards Rural Prosperity. Department of animal husbandry, livestock fisheries and veterinary services, Government of Sikkim. Retrieved from http://www.sikkim-ahvs.gov.in/pdf/ALL%20IN%20ONE.pdf on 15-09-20.

Anonymous. (2018). Cattle and dairy development. Department of animal husbandry, dairying and fisheries, Ministry of agriculture and farmers welfare, Government of India. Retrieved from http://dahd.nic.in/about-us/divisions/cattle-and-dairy-development on 10-09-2020

Anonymous. (2018). ENVIS Sikkim: Status of Environment and Related Issues. Forest and Environment Department, Government of Sikkim. Retrieved from http://sikenvis.nic.in/Database/Agriculture_777.aspx#:~:text=The%20economy%20of%20Sikkim%20is,security%20of%20sizeable%20native%20population.&text=It%20is%20estimated%20that%20over,%2C%20food%2C%20and%20nutritional%20security on 15-01-21.

Anonymous. (2019). 20th Livestock Census. Basic Animal Husbandry, Department of animal husbandry, dairying and fisheries, Ministry of agriculture and farmers welfare, Government of India. Retrieved from http://www.dahd.nic.in/ on 19-02-21.

Anonymous. (2019). State dairy profile. Department of animal husbandry, dairying and fisheries, Ministry of agriculture and farmers welfare, Government of India. Retrieved from http://dahd.nic.in/about-us/divisions/cattle-and-dairy-development on 20-12-20

Anonymous. (2021). Department of animal husbandry, livestock, fisheries & veterinary services, Government of Sikkim. Retrieved from https://southsikkim.nic.in/departments/animal-husbandry-livestock-fisheries-veterinary on 15-08-2020

Badole, R. (2006). A study on knowledge and adoption of improved dairy practices by dairy co-operative society members of Ashta Block of Sehore district, Madhya Pradesh. *M.Sc. (Ag) Thesis (Unpublished),* R.A.K. College of Agriculture, Sehore.

Basha, S. K. (2017). An empirical study on rural women empowerment through self- help groups and providing various earning opportunities in rural villages in Prakasam district, Andhra Pradesh. *International Journal of Scientific and Research Publication.* **7**(7):553-566.

Batool, S. A. and Jadoon, A. K. (2018). Women's empowerment and associated age-related factors. *Pakistan Journal of Social and Clinical Psychology.* **16**(2): 52-56.

Bhanotra, A., Wankhade, V., Khandey, S. A. and Kumar, P. (2015). Role of rural women in decision making process regarding livestock management. *Journal of Animal Research.* **5**(3): 555-559.

Bharathamma, G. U. (2005). Empowerment of rural women through income generating activities in Gadag district of North Karnataka. *M. Sc. (Agri.) Thesis (Unpublished),* UAS, Dharwad-58000.

Bhasin, M. K., and Bhasin, V. (1995). Sikkim Himalayas: Ecology and Resources Development, Kamla- Raj Enterprise. New Delhi.

Bose, D. K, Srivastava, J. P. and Masih, E. (2013). Participation of women in livestock management activities in Cooch Behar district of West Bengal. *Indian Journal of Extension Education.* **49**(1&2): 40-42.

Chakravarthi, M. K., Krishna, M. B., Satya, N. and Sreedhar, S. (2017). Constraints of dairy farming in Kadapa district of Andhra Pradesh. *Indian Journal of Animal Production and Management.* **33**(1/2): 7-10.

Chauhan, N. M. (2011). Role performance of tribal farm women in domestic and agricultural activities in Gujarat state. *Journal of Progressive Agriculture.* **2**(3):21-27.

Chinnadurai, S., Chinnadsurai, P. and Markanday, J. C. (2002). Farm women in commercial dairy farming. *Journal of Dairying Foods and Home Sciences.* **21**(1):63-65.

Damodar, P. P., Shaikh, J. I. and Mali, M. D. (2016). Relationship of personal, socio-economic and situational characteris*tics with the empowerment of rural* w**o**men. Agriculture update. 11(1):93-95.

Damodar, P and Radhod, M. K. (2013). Empowerment of rural women through the activities of Mahila Arthik Vikas Mahamandal. Indian Journa*l of Applied Resea*rc**h.** 3(8):4-6.

Das, J. K., Bhattacharjee, S., Datta, J., Mazumder, G. and Laskar, T. (2019). Influence of Socio-economic Factors on Empowerment of Farm Women: An In-Depth Analysis. *International Journal of Current Microbiology and Applied Science.* **8**(07): 967-977.

Dash, S. Sarangi, M. K., Dash, M., Sahoo, D. S. and Muduli, K. (2020). Role of dairy cooperative society in empowering women in rural Odisha. *International Journal of Advanced Science and Technology.* **29**(7):461-467.

Devi, Y. L. (2016). Exploring the Involvement of Women in Dairy Farming as An Alternative Livelihood in Manipur. *M.Sc. (AGRI.) Thesis (Unpublished),* UBKV Cooch Behar, (WB)

Dhayal, B. L. and Mehta, B. M. (2020). Constraints perceived by the tribal farm women in acquiring training on animal husbandry practices in Chhotaudepur district of Gujarat. *Journal of Krishi Vigyan.* **8**(2):45-48.

Fatima, S. and Akhtar, M. W. (2014). Empowerment of Rural Women through Dairy Industry in Begusarai District, Bihar. *International Journal of Application or Innovation in Engineering and Management.* **3**(10):130-133.

Gunjkar, V. P. (2005). Empowerment opportunities of farm women in Gorwhar village under IVLP. *M.Sc. (Agri.) Thesis (Unpublished)*, Dr. PDKV, Akola.

Gupta, A., Saha, A., Gupta, R. K., Chakraborty, S., and Dhakre D. S. (2020). Socio-economic status of rural women dairy farmers in Surguja district of Chhattisgarh. *Bulletin of Environment, Pharmacology and Life Sciences.* **9**(4):112-116.

Hasan, M. M., Kabir, S. M., and Kader, A. M. (2020). Enhancing resilience through women empowerment and livestock production in selected area of Satkhira district of Bangladesh. *Journal of Entrepreneurship and Business Resilience.* **3**(2):53-72.

Hundal, J. S., Singh, P., Bhatti, J. S. and Kansal, S. K. (2015). Constraints faced by farmers in adoption of dairy as entrepreneurship. *Haryana Veterinarian.* **54**(1):67-69.

Islam, M. R., Kabir, S. M. L. and Islam, M. S. (2019). Women's empowerment through small-scale dairy farming in Bangladesh: A study on some selected areas of Mymensingh district. *Asian-Australian Journal of Food Safety and Security.* **3**(2):85-95.

Islam, M. S., Ahmed, M. F. and Alam, M. S. (2014). The role of microcredit program on women empowerment: Empirical evidence from rural Bangladesh. *Developing Country Studies.* **4**(5):90-97.

Jadav, S. J., Rani, V. D., Mudgal, S. and Dhamsaniya, H. B. (2014). Women empowerment through training in dairy farming. *Asian Journal of Dairy and Food Research.* **33**(2): 147-153.

Jahan, N. and Khan, N. (2016). To study the participation of farm women in various agriculture and allied activities. *International Journal of Home Science.* **2**(2):180-186.

Javed, A., Sadaf, S. and Luqman, M. (2006). Rural women's participation in crop and livestock production activities in Faisalabad, Pakistan. *Journal of Agriculture and Social science.* **2** (3): 150-154.

Kabeer, N. (1999). Resources, agency, achievements: Reflections on the measurement of women's empowerment. *Development and Change.* **30**(3): 435-464.

Kadam, R. P., Umate, S.M., Pawar, G.S. and Nair, R.G. (2014). Empowerment of women through self-help group in Marathwada region. *International Journal of Home Science Extension and Communication and Management.***1**(2):127-133.

Kale, R. A., Tekale, V. S. and Gaikwad, J. H. (2013). Constraints faced by farm women in dairy farming. *Research Journal of Animal Husbandry and Dairy Science.* **4**(2):58-60.

Kamalkannan, K. and Namasivayam, N. (2005). Economic empowerment of women through entrepreneurship development. *Kisan World.* **32**(9):26-28.

Kathiriya, J. B., Damasia, D. M. and Kabaria, B. B. (2013). Role of rural women in dairy farming of Rajkot district. *Tamil Nadu Journal of Veterinary & Animal Sciences.* **9**(4):239-247.

Kaur, K. (2015). Participation of rural women in dairy activities. *Journal of Krishi Vigyan.* **4**(1):72-75.

Kaur, M., Mishra, B., Singh, P., Singh, A. and Rathore, S. (2011). Measurement of empowerment extent of rural women. *Pantnagar Journal of Research.* **9**(1):138-140.

Kaur, P, Kaur, L. and Astha. (2021). Status of rural women in dairy farming in Amritsar district of Punjab. *Asian Journal of Agricultural Extension, Economics and Sociology.* **39**(5):106-113.

Kaur, S., Singh, J., Verma, H. K., Dash, S. K. and Kansal, S. K. (2019). Participation appraisal of women farmers in dairy husbandry practices in Indo-Pak border area of Punjab (India). *International Journal of Current Microbiology and Applied Sciences.* **8**(05):2298-2305.

Kaushal, S. K. and Singh, Y.K. (2010). Socio-economic correlates of women empowerment. *Indian Research Journal of Extension Education.* **10**(2): 81-84.

Kavithaa, N. V. and Rajkumar, N. V. (2016). Decision making behaviour of farm women in dairy farming activities in Erode district of Tamil Nadu. *International Journal of Science, Environment and Technology.* **5**(2): 416-419.

Khan, M., Sajjad, M., Hameed, B., Khan, M. N. and Jan, A. U. (2012). Participation of women in agriculture activities in district Peshawar. *Sarhad Journal of Agriculture*. **28**(1):121-127.

Khan, N., Parashari, A. K. and Salman, M. S. (2014). Role of dairy cooperatives in socio-economic Development of dairy farmers in Moradabad district: A case study. *International Journal of Social Sciences*. **2**(1): 1-8.

Khan, T. M. and Maan, A. A. (2008). Socio-culture milieu of women's empowerment in district Faisalabad. *Pakistan Journal of Agricultural Science*. **45**(3):78-90

Narmatha, N., Uma, V., Arun, L. and Geetha, R. (2009). Level of participation of women in livestock farming activities. *Tami Nadu Journal of Veterinary Science*. **5**(1):4-8.

Niketha, L., Sankhala, G., Kumar, S. and Prasad, K. (2018). Constraints faced by the members of women dairy cooperatives in Karnataka, India. *International Journal of Current Microbiology and Applied Sciences*. **7**(5):977-985.

Nithya, P. and Selvaraj, R. (2018). An analysis of constraints faced by the farmers in rearing buffaloes in Tirupur district of Tamil Nadu. *International Journals of Science, Environment and Technology*. (5):1655-1661.

Panchbhai, G. J., Siddiqui, M. F., Sawant, M. N., Verma, A. P. and Parmeswaranaik, J. (2017). Constraints faced by cooperative dairy farmers in adoption of recommended dairy management practices. *International Journal of Current Microbiology and Applied Sciences*. **6**(3): 1962-1966.

Patel, K., Chaudhary, G. M., Ghasura, R. S. and Aswar, B. K. (2015). Constraints faced by dairy farm women in improved animal husbandry practices of Banaskantha district of North Gujarat. *Indian Journal of Hill farming*. **28**(2):130-132.

Patel, S. J., Kumar, R., Patel, A. S., Patel, N. R. and Parmar, V. N. (2017). Involvement of farm women in decision making regarding dairy farming in Junagadh district of Gujarat state. *Indian Journal of Hill Farming*. **30**(1): 45-58.

Patel, S. J., Kumar, R., Patel, M. D., Patel, A. S. and Patel, N. R. (2016). Constraints faced by the farm women in dairy farming in Junagadh district of Gujarat State, India. *Life Sciences Leaflets*.**79**: 27-33.

Pathade, S. S., Sawant, M. N., Ramesh, N., Pordhiya, K. I. and Sadashive, S. M. (2017). Constraints faced by women self-help groups involved in dairy farming from Hingoli district of Maharashtra. *Indian Journal of Extension Education*. **53**(4):129-131.

Prasad, K., Savale, S., Mahantesh, M. T., Pavan, M., Barman, D. and Abraham, J. (2017). Socio-economic profile and constraints faced by dairy farmers of Wayanad district, India. *International Journal of Current Microbiology and Applied Sciences*. **6**(6):870-874.

Rahman, M. H., & Naoroze, K. (2007). Women empowerment through participation in aquaculture: Experience of a large-scale technology demonstration project in Bangladesh. *FAO, Agris* retrieved: https://agris.fao.org/agris-search/search.do?recordID=AV20120141579 on 15-2-2021.

Rao, E. K. (2006). Role of Women in Agriculture: A Micro Level Study. *Journal of Global Economy*. **2**(2): 107-118.

Rathod, P. K., Nikam, T. R., Landge, S., Vajreshwari, S. and Hatey, A. (2011). Participation of rural women in dairy farming in Karnataka. *Indian Research Journal of Extension Education*. **11**(2):31-36.

Redzuan, M., Nikkhah, H. A., and Abu-Samah, A. (2010). The Effect of Women's Socio-demographic Variables on their Empowerment. *Journal of American Science*. **6**(11):426-434.

Sadashive, S. M., Pathade, S. S., Pordhiya, K. I. and Ramesh, N. (2016). Constraints perceived by the dairy farmers in running dairy enterprises. *International Journal of Science, Environment and Technology*. **5**(5):3120-3124.

Sajesh, V. K., Ramasundaram, P. and Singh, P. (2011). Impact of self-help groups on empowerment of rural women: A Case of Kudumbasree programme in Kerala. *Indian Journal of Extension Education*. **47**(3&4): 14-19.

Sampat, K. K. (2008). Empowerment of rural women through self help group. *M.Sc. (Agri.) Thesis (Unpublished)*, Dr. PDKV, Akola.

Shambharkar, Y. B., Jadhav, U. V. and Mankar, D. M. (2012). Impact of self- help groups on empowerment of women member. *Indian Research Journal of Extension Education*. **2**(Special issue):188-192.

Shankar, R., Sharma, A., Jha, G. and Negi, B. (2017). A study on constraints faced by sampled dairy respondents in adoption of improved dairy management practices. *Progressive Research- An International Journal*. **12**(1):33-35.

Shanti, S and Murty, A. V. N. (2019). Impact of socio economic determinants on women empowerment in India (Working women in selected districts of Andhra Pradesh). *International Journal of Engineering and Advanced Technology*. **8**(3S):458-462.

Sharma, A. (2008). A study on role of farm women in agriculture operation and decision-making pattern in Sanchi bock of Raisen district of Madhya Pradesh. *M.Sc. (Agri.) (Unpublished),* JNKVV, Jabalpur (M.P.)

Sharma, A., Kumar, S. and Kandpal, N. K. (2018). Constraints faced by the dairy farm women: A study in Nainital District of Uttarakhand, India. *Indian Research Journal of Extension Education*. **18**(2):86-90.

Sheikh, Q. A., Meraj, M. and Sadaqat, M. (2016). Gender equality and socio-economic development through women's empowerment in Pakistan. *Ritsumeikan Journal of Asia Pacific Studies*. **34**:142-160.

Shiralashetti, A. S. (2013). Economic empowerment of women entrepreneurs-A study of district of North Karnataka. *International Journal of Multidisciplinary Management Studies*. **3**(7):45-57.

Singh, P., Rampal, V. K., Sharma, K. and Dhaliwal, N. S. (2019). Constraint analysis of dairy farmers in Malwa region of Punjab. *Journal of Community Mobilization and Sustainable Development*. **14**(3):384-388.

Singh, V., Rewani, S. K., Rajoria, S. K., and Saini, G. R. (2017). Constraints faced by women dairy cooperative society members in Jaipur, Rajasthan, India. *International Journal of Current Microbiology and Applied Sciences*. **6**(12):2612-2618.

Sudhindra, H. R. (2005). Empowerment through watershed development. *Social Welfare*. **53**(3): 16-17.

Tayde, V. (2006). Empowerment of rural women in Marathwada region of Maharashtra State. *Ph.D. Thesis (Unpublished)*, M.A.U. Parbhani.

Tayde, V. V. and Chole, R. R. (2010). Empowerment appraisal of rural women in Marathwada Region of Maharashtra State. *Indian Research Journal of Extension Education*. **10(**1): 33-36.

Tekale, V. S., Jadhav, J. D. and Shaikh, J. I. (2014). Empowerment of rural women through self help group. *International Journal of Extension Education*.**10**:60-64.

Thakur, D. and Chandar, M. (2006). Gender based differential access to information among Livestock owners and its impact on household milk production in Kangra district of Himachal Pradesh. *Indian Journal of Dairy Science*. **59**(6):401-404.

Toppo, A., Trivedinand, M. S. and Patel, A. (2004). Participation of farm women in dairy occupation. *Gujarat Journal of Extension Education*. **15**(2):15-21.

Upadhyay, M. and Yadav, C. M. (2015). Involvement of members and non -members of women dairy cooperatives in dairy husbandry activities. *Indian Journal of Animal Production and Management.* **31**(1/2):4-7.

Upadhyay, S., Kaur, M. and Desai, C. P. (2013). Constraints analysis of dairy farm women in animal husbandry. *Journal of Progressive Agriculture.* **4**(2):63-67.

Verma, S. K, (1992). Women in agriculture: A socio economic analysis. Concept publishing company, A15-16, Commercial building, Mohan Garden, New Delhi.

Yadav, K. D. K. and Revanna, M. L. (2017). A study on socio-economic status of the farm women of Tumakuru district of Karnataka state, India. *International Journal of Pure and Applied Bioscience.* **5**(4):309-314.

Yadav, S. and Sethi, N. (2000). Gain in knowledge among dairy women through media. *Maharashtra Journal of Extension Education.* **2**(19):277-279.

Yasmin, S. and Ikemoto, Y. (2015). Women's participation in small scale dairy farming for poverty reduction in Bangladesh. *American International Journal of Social Science.* **4**(5):21-33.

Younas, M., S. Gulrez and H. Rehman. (2007). Women's role in livestock production. The Dawn, December 17. https://www.dawn.com/news/280622 retrieved on 17-09-2020.

www.mapsofindia.com

# 8

# Appendix

***Interview Schedule***

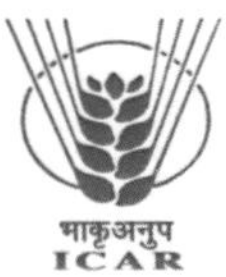


**ICAR-NATIONAL DAIRY RESEARCH INSTITUTE**

**(Deemed University)**

**Karnal, Haryana**

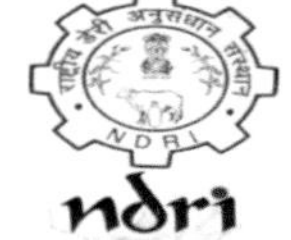


**Title: Retrospective multidimensional study on magnitude of participation of women in dairying farming in East district of Sikkim"**

**Interview Schedule for primary data collection**

- Name of the respondent:
- Village name:
- Block name:
- Mobile number:
- Respondent id:

## A. Socio-personal information

| 1. | Age: | | |
|---|---|---|---|
| 2. | Education: | Illiterate (0) | |
| | | Primary school (1) | |
| | | Secondary school (2) | |
| | | Higher sec. school (3) | |
| | | Graduate and above (4) | |
| 3. | Marital status: | Married | |
| | | Unmarried | |
| | | Widow | |
| 4. | Family type: | Nuclear (0) | |
| | | Joint (1) | |
| 5. | Family size: | Small family (Up to 4) (0): | |
| | | Large family (above 4) (1): | |
| 6. | Farming experience in years: | | |
| 7. | Social status | (Gen (1)/OBC (2) /SC (3)/ST (4): | |

8. Occupation

| | | |
|---|---|---|
| 1. | Agriculture farming (0) | |
| 2. | Agri +Dairy farming (1) | |
| 3. | Dairy farming (2) | |
| 4. | Labor work +Agri +dairy farming (3) | |
| 5. | Other (please specify) (4) | |

9. Land holding

| | | |
|---|---|---|
| 1. | Marginal (<1 ha) (0) | |
| 2. | Small (1 to 2 ha) (1) | |

10. Annual income through dairying ..........................

11. Herd size:

| | | | |
|---|---|---|---|
| 1. | Cow | Milch | |
| | | Dry | |
| 2. | Bull | | |
| 3. | Total | | |

12. production per day……liters

14. Asset possession

| | | |
|---|---|---|
| 1. | Land possession | |
| 2. | Building | |
| 3. | Farm machineries(specify) | |
| 4. | Insurance/ Bonds | |
| 5. | Others | |

15. Livestock possession

| **Sl. No** | **Livestock** | | **Total** |
|---|---|---|---|
| 1. | Cow | Local | |
| | | Exotic | |
| 2. | Buffalo | | |
| 3. | Sheep | | |
| 4. | Pig | | |
| 5. | Goat | | |
| 6. | Poultry | | |

16. Access to finance

| 1. | Bank | |
|---|---|---|
| 2. | Friends/ Relatives | |
| 3. | Self Help Group | |
| 4. | Village head | |

17. Social Participation:

| Sl. No | Institute | Member | |
|---|---|---|---|
| | | Participation | No Participation |
| 1. | Gram panchayat | | |
| 2. | Cooperative society | | |
| 3. | Self -help groups | | |
| 4. | Anganwadi | | |
| 5. | Religious group | | |
| 6. | Other (please specify) | | |

18. Source of information

| Sl.No | Sources | Every time (4) | Often (3) | Sometime (2) | Never (1) |
|---|---|---|---|---|---|
| 1. | Radio | | | | |
| 2. | Newspaper | | | | |
| 3. | Television | | | | |
| 4. | Training program | | | | |
| 5. | VLW | | | | |
| 6. | Extension personal | | | | |
| 7. | KVK | | | | |
| 8. | Agriculture officers | | | | |
| 9. | Veterinary officers | | | | |

19. Time utilization pattern:

| Sl.No | Activities | Time/day |
|---|---|---|
| 1. | Collection of fodder | |
| 2. | Preparation of feed and feeding | |
| 3. | Cleaning of animal and cow shed | |
| 4. | Milking of the cattle | |
| 6. | Selling of milk | |

## Part 1

**Objective 1:** To assess the differential role accomplished by women dairy farmers from different social strata in the study area.

| Sl.No | Activities | Regularly (4) | Often (3) | Sometimes (2) | Never (1) |
|---|---|---|---|---|---|
| **A.** | **Breeding aspect** | | | | |
| 1. | Choosing different breeds of cattle | | | | |
| 2. | Contacting veterinarian officials for A. I. | | | | |
| 3. | Taking animal for natural service | | | | |
| 4. | Consulting veterinarian for infertility management | | | | |
| **B.** | **Feeding aspect** | | | | |
| 1. | Collection of feed and fodder | | | | |
| 2. | Feeding the animal | | | | |
| 3. | Storage of feed and fodder | | | | |
| 4. | Watering and feed supplement | | | | |
| **D.** | **Marketing aspect** | | | | |
| 1. | Selling of milk and milk products to the household | | | | |
| 2. | Selling of milk to cooperatives | | | | |
| 3. | Selling of value-added products | | | | |
| **E.** | **Health care Aspect** | | | | |
| 1. | Care of diseased animal | | | | |
| 2. | Care of pregnant cows | | | | |
| 3. | Care of new born calf | | | | |
| 4. | Vaccination management | | | | |
| 5. | Deforming management | | | | |
| **F.** | **Housing Aspect** | | | | |
| 1. | Cleaning of the cattle shed | | | | |
| 2. | Construction of cattle shed | | | | |
| 3. | Use of dung for manure | | | | |
| 4. | Cleaning of animal before milking | | | | |
| 5. | Milking of animal | | | | |
| 6. | Record keeping | | | | |
| **H.** | **Economic aspect** | | | | |
| 1. | Taking loans for dairy cattle | | | | |
| 2. | Insurance of the animals | | | | |
| 3. | Sale of the cattle | | | | |

| | | | | | |
|---|---|---|---|---|---|
| 4. | Purchase of cattle | | | | |
| **I.** | **Decision making aspect** | | | | |
| 1. | Expansion of the farm | | | | |
| 2. | Adopting new farm technologies | | | | |
| 3. | Preparation of milk products | | | | |

**Objective 2:** To measure the magnitude of socio-economic empowerment of women dairy farmer of the study area.

| Sl.No | Parameters | Responses | |
|---|---|---|---|
| **I.** | **Social Dimension** | Yes | No |
| 1. | Do you participate in local club committee meeting without any hinderance? | | |
| 2. | Whether you put forward your opinions related to any injustice in the public? | | |
| 3. | Are you allowed to work outside the home to earn income? | | |
| 4. | Whether you are allowed to interact with unknown person at public places? | | |
| 5. | Whether you get the feeling of social appreciation in the society? | | |
| 6. | Do you caste vote independently? | | |
| 7. | Are you allowed to do your choice of work? | | |
| 8. | Do you have freedom to socialize with your friends? | | |
| 9. | Do you feel satisfied with your social status? | | |
| 10. | Whether you have access to cereals @ 300g/day throughout the year? | | |
| 11. | Whether you have daily access to pulses @ 90g/day throughout the year? | | |
| 12. | Whether you have daily access to vegetables @300g/day throughout the year? | | |
| 13. | Whether you have daily access to milk @300g/day throughout the year? | | |
| 14. | Whether you have daily access to fruits @150g/day throughout the year? | | |
| **II.** | **Economic Dimension** | | |
| 1. | Are you having saving bank account in your name? | | |
| 2. | Do you have fixed deposit in your name? | | |
| 3. | Do you have insurance in your name? | | |
| 4. | Whether you have liberty to spend on personal belongings? | | |
| 5. | Do you save money from the household income? | | |
| 6. | Do you have independence to purchase household appliances? | | |
| 7. | Do you have the authority to hire labor? | | |
| **III.** | **"Freedom to mobility" Dimension** | | |
| 1. | Do you have liberty to visit hospitals for health checkup? | | |
| 2. | Do you have autonomy to visit hospitals for children's health checkup? | | |
| 3. | Do you have the liberty to visit your friends when you have some work with them? | | |

| | | | |
|---|---|---|---|
| 4. | Do you have the independence to visit your maternal family whenever you feel needed? | | |
| 5. | Do you have restrictions to visit relatives and neighbors? | | |
| 6. | Do you have the free will to attend marriage ceremonies? | | |
| 7. | Do you have the autonomy to travel from one place alone? | | |
| 8. | Do you independently visit new places? | | |
| 9. | Whether you have freedom to go for grocery shopping at market? | | |
| 10. | Do you visit religious places? | | |
| 11. | Whether you have liberty to visit institutional credit sources? | | |
| 12. | Do you visit different place to attend training programme by yourself? | | |
| **IV.** | **"Technical knowledge possession" Dimension** | | |
| 1. | Do you have access to internet on you mobile? | | |
| 2. | Do you have access to social media information? | | |
| 3. | Are you comfortable in using electronic gadgets? | | |
| 4. | Do you have access to information on different government schemes for promoting dairy development? | | |
| **V.** | **Decision making Dimension** | | |
| 1. | Do you take decision in availing loans from the bank? | | |
| 2. | Do you take decision in day to day buying of household items? | | |
| 3. | Do you take decision in saving of income? | | |
| 4. | Do you take decision in acceptance of innovative technology? | | |
| 5. | Do you take decision in schooling of children? | | |
| 6. | Do you take decision in birth control? | | |
| 7. | Do you take decision in starting a new enterprise? | | |

**Objective 3:** To analyze the feedback of women engaged in dairying. Please rank the statements according to the order of your importance.

| Sl.No | Feedbacks | Rank | Suggestion |
|---|---|---|---|
| **A.** | **Economical aspect** | | |
| 1. | High cost of crossbred animal | | |
| 2. | High cost of concentrate feed and fodder | | |
| 3. | Difficulty in getting loans from bank | | |
| 4. | Lack of schemes for purchasing milch cattle | | |
| 5. | High cost of medicine for cattle | | |
| 6. | Low productivity of local breed | | |
| 7. | Lack of transport facility for milk and animal. | | |
| **B.** | **Technical aspects** | | |
| 1. | Lack of bulk milk cooler in the milk centre | | |
| 2. | Lack of machine milking system | | |
| 3. | Lack of training on scientific cattle management. | | |
| 4. | Lack of awareness on disease management | | |
| 5. | Delayed service of animal health officials | | |
| 6. | Problem in heat detection | | |
| **C.** | **Administrative aspects** | | |
| 1. | Lack of financial support from govt. | | |
| 2. | Lack of veterinary service in the village | | |
| 3. | Lack of schemes promoting dairy farming | | |
| 4. | Lack of training availability on new technology to the farmers | | |
| 5. | Lack of extension contacts in the village | | |
| **D.** | **Information networking aspect** | | |
| 1. | Irregular information on govt. schemes on dairy | | |
| 2. | Lack of information on new technology | | |
| 3. | Lack of information on training of dairy practices | | |
| 4. | Lack of information on disease and pest management | | |
| 5. | Irregular information on AI | | |
| **E.** | **Independence decision making aspect** | | |
| 1. | Non availability of financial support | | |
| 2. | Lack of knowledge on dairy activities | | |
| 3. | Poor managerial skills | | |
| 4. | Lack of self-confidence | | |
| | | | |

# Index